Healthy in Seven Days

Dr. med. Raimund von Helden

Healthy in Seven Days

Success through vitamin D treatment

A practical guide

Hygeia publishing

Disclaimer

This book has been put together with care. However, the author and publisher bear no liability for the accuracy of any information or recommendations, or for any printing errors. Please consult your doctor if you have any complaints or illnesses.

Library and Archives Cataloguing in Publication Data

Raimund von Helden: *Healthy in Seven Days. Success through vitamin D treatment. A practical guide. Symptoms, Validation, Remedy.*
Hygeia publishing Dresden 2014.

Printed in Germany

Editor: Thomas Klein

ISBN 978-3-939865-21-6

www.hygeia-publishing.com
www.vitamindelta.org

Nobody will be able to cure diseases
unless they know the causes.

AURELIUS CORNELIUS CELSUS

Contents

Acknowledgments

I would like to thank my wife Maria and our three children for their crucial assistance with the project; Mr. Thomas Klein from Hygeia publishing for his clear plans and tireless expert support; my associate Dr. Stephan Moenninghoff for his cooperation; Professor Armin Zittermann (Bad Oeynhausen) for his friendly advice; Professor Joerg Reichrath (Homburg, Saar) for his warm welcome; Professor Joerg Spitz (Schlangenbad) for his activities; Dr. William B. Grant (San Francisco, USA) for his explicit answers to my many questions; Professor Michael F. Holick (Boston, USA) for his professional suggestions and encouragement; Professor Reinhold Vieth (Toronto, Canada) for his explanations; members of the international *Vitamin D Research Group* and all those who support the *VitaminDelta* project.

About the author

Dr. med. Raimund von Helden has been a doctor since 1984 – and has worked at a joint practice for general medicine in Lennestadt (Germany) since 1991. In this book, he reports on his successes in treating acute vitamin D deficiency, and on the importance of vitamin D for restoring and preserving our health.

The author looks forward to hearing readers' responses, and welcomes suggestions and criticism. He can be contacted at www.vitaminDelta.org

Foreword

In his book *Healthy in Seven Days*, Dr. Raimund von Helden examines the use of Vitamin D to treat many illnesses. The MANOS concept (Muscles, Adynamia, Nervous system, Orthostasis, Skeletal damage) covers the main symptoms of acute vitamin D deficiency. The book contains many informative case studies, showing how these complaints and illnesses can be permanently remedied by eliminating the cause.

Vitamin D deficiency is a widespread issue nowadays, and one of the main causes of disease in many patients. Science has shown that an optimum vitamin D level is over 40 ng/ml. The risk of infections, heart disease and cancer drops significantly in this range, while life expectancy increases.

Anyone wanting to regain health, joie de vivre and creativeness, and maintain these in old age, should heed the information presented in this book.

William B. Grant, Ph.D. – San Francisco, June 2011
Author of of more than 180 scientific articles on vitamin D, and the founding director of the *Sunlight, Nutrition And Health Research Center* – www.sunarc.org

A surprise after twenty years as a doctor

I had been working as a doctor for twenty years when I first measured the vitamin D content in a patient's blood in 2005: The reading fell below the measurability threshold of 7 ng/ml. I felt guilty, because, until then, I had been unable to provide this patient with the correct treatment, even though vitamin D was available at low cost.

Thereafter, barely a day passed when I didn't encounter a patient with a serious deficiency. Vitamin D deficiency proved to be a mass phenomenon. It is the most common pathological laboratory result in Germany, as well as in other industrialized countries. It is staggering that this matter had gone undetected in medical practices for so long, even though the scientific findings are loud and clear.

Optimum vitamin D levels cannot be achieved with freely available vitamin D or multivitamin formulae. The required dose is much too low for this. The general recommendations for vitamin D intake cannot fix deficiency; even good vitamin D levels cannot be maintained. I thus increased vitamin D intake until my patients reached the same optimum level found in the indigenous people of sun-blessed countries.

Incredible success can be achieved when an optimum vitamin D level is reached: nut, apple and animal hair allergies disappeared, migraines decreased, dizziness fits with auditory defects (Menière's disease) were eliminated, chronic back pain dissipated, patient attitude improved, and there were no signs of calf cramps, sun allergies or long-lasting weariness. Many cases of chronic fatigue and depression improved after just one week, though bone pain took longer to heal, sometimes even a few months.

Vitamin D therapy is affordable, easy and low-risk. A vitamin D deficiency can be accurately diagnosed and quickly rectified using a natural substance. Every doctor should incorporate vitamin D therapy into his/her practice, because many patients suffer from a serious deficiency - both in summer, and even more so in winter. There is no alternative to vitamin D therapy; it is the only way to eliminate the cause of the resulting illnesses.

Vitamin D therapy can be administered using medication or radiation. In the case of the former, specific doses can be prescribed, enabling an optimum vitamin D level to be reached within just a few days. Radiation takes longer to replenish stores and reach an optimum level – usually around two months, even with high altitude treatment.

Light therapy is a very old practice, having achieved success even in ancient times. Hippocrates himself recommended daily sunbathing.

People still underestimate the amount of vitamin D the body actually needs. We have to go by the levels found in the indigenous peoples of the tropics, which is the only way to maintain good health in the long term.

It is astonishing that, as a result of official monitoring, animals in Germany have better access to vitamin D than humans do.

The book's title *Healthy in Seven Days* seeks to explain that rectifying a vitamin D deficiency often also allows other illnesses to suddenly disappear, even if the patients have been suffering from them for years. However, these successes can only be achieved if doses are high enough to ensure an optimum vitamin D level can be reached and maintained.

This book presents the complaints and illnesses suspected to be caused by a vitamin D deficiency. It aims to help readers become more aware of vitamin D, and get a better idea about the many different symptoms of a deficiency, which are often left untreated for years due to their unknown cause. Case studies allow readers to see the effectiveness of vitamin D therapy for themselves.

Up to eighty percent of deficiency patients notice an improvement as a result of the vitamin D therapy. If there is no improvement in health, it means the symptoms are due to other illnesses whose causes should be determined. But even these patients benefit from having their vitamin D increased to an optimum level: Their overall health improves, their cancer risk drops, and their life expectancy increases, since a vitamin D deficiency significantly increases the risk of cancer, diabetes mellitus, multiple sclerosis, autoimmune diseases, osteoporosis, arteriosclerosis, and high blood pressure.

Symptoms of vitamin D deficiency

A young man came slowly into my consulting room. He was complaining that he could no longer do his work at his company. “I’m totally washed up. Everything hurts, I’m exhausted, and can’t sleep properly. It’s been getting worse and worse over the last few weeks.”

He had not taken a sunny vacation in three years. He was smoking a packet of cigarettes a day. Upon rectifying his vitamin D deficiency, he was restored to good health within three days.

Undetected vitamin D deficiency

If you are kept up all night coughing, you generally go to see the doctor the next day. On the other hand, there are numerous symptoms which are so subtle and inconspicuous that many people hesitate for a long time before finally consulting a doctor. Hardly anyone goes to the doctor and says, “I have fitful sleep, calf cramps, and am always tired.” Which is why people suffering from a vitamin D deficiency only go to the doctor very late, by chance, or not at all.

Doctors often dismiss these symptoms as “mentally-based functional disorders of the emotional state”. “It’s all in your mind” – patients are initially relieved to hear this comment, but it also means they are left on their own, helpless. Many patients suspect the doctor won’t be able to help them with their problems, so they refrain from mentioning them.

It is no coincidence that these symptoms are disregarded in university medicine. Only GPs who come into contact with an unfiltered horde of patients on a daily basis know how common these disorders really are.

"Take a vacation!" This well-meant medical advice enables a vitamin D deficiency to be highlighted as possible causes of illness. But very few patients can actually heed this advice and end up enjoying a vacation in the sun.

Typical complaints caused by a vitamin D deficiency

Acute vitamin D deficiencies can usually be rectified very quickly. Illnesses caused by chronic vitamin D deficiencies, on the other hand, take longer to cure. In many cases they may even be incurable due to the resulting degenerative damage. This particularly relates to bone deformity in the event of osteomalacia (softening of the bone, known as rickets in children), as well as broken vertebrae and bone damage caused by advanced osteoporosis.

This book deals with acute vitamin D deficiency, whose typical symptoms can be split into five groups:

- *M – Muscle disorders*: Muscle cramps, twitches, trembling, vibrating, pain and muscle weakness.
- *A – Adynamic disorders*: Debility, listlessness, lack of energy, permanent exhaustion and constant fatigue.
- *N – Nervous system disorders*: Dizziness, paresthesia, sleep disorders, sudden awakening, a great need for sleep, impaired concentration, restlessness, anxiety, behavioral changes such as aggression, impaired coordination and vertigo, instability when walking and standing.
- *O – Orthostatic disorders*: Circulatory disorders, daily headaches increasing at noon, feeling cold, freezing, especially in hands and feet at night time, Raynaud syndrome.
- *S – Skeletal disorders*: Pain in bones and joints increasing with exercise, reduction in bone mass and tendency to suffer fractures, bones painful to the touch.

The first letter of each of these five aspects on vitamin D deficiency forms the acronym of the new syndrome: M-A-N-O-S. These five signs have been puzzling so far, but can be easily understood.

Muscular dysfunction. – Serious vitamin D deficiency often results in eyelid twitches and twitches in arm and leg muscles, as well as vibrating muscle fibers (fasciculations), cramps and muscular pain, particularly at night. Soles of the feet can cramp up, and neck muscles may be tense. A vitamin D deficiency can also lead to weakened myocardial muscles.

How can these symptoms be explained? Muscle function requires a sufficient supply of calcium, because muscle cell contractions are triggered by an inflow of calcium. If calcium is lacking due to a vitamin D deficiency, the body has to save it, providing less calcium for the muscles, especially at night. This particularly explains the appearance of symptoms at night, e.g. the typical pain in leg muscles. An improvement is generally achieved within seven days.

Adynamia. – A healthy person is dynamic; they enjoy exercise and activity, while a sick person is adynamic, suffering from weakness, exhaustion and listlessness (chronic fatigue). These patients need a lot of sleep, but are never properly refreshed or energized, even after a long sleep.

Medical textbooks dedicate entire chapters to this phenomenon, yet the most likely cause, vitamin D deficiency, is never mentioned.

We associate the term chalk with dead stone. And the name of the trace element calcium is derived from this. But it is highly reactive. If pure calcium is placed in water, it triggers a fierce chemical reaction with fizzing and vapor.

The calcium ions in the body are equivalent to the ignition

voltage in a combustion engine. If this voltage is reduced, the combustion process slows. Low vitamin D levels disrupt the calcium supply, meaning calcium must be released sparingly. This makes it difficult to activate the muscle cells, causing over-exertion of muscles and, in extreme cases, debilitating weariness.

Symptoms are usually more intense at night, but may also cause problems by day if the deficiency is particularly severe. Adynamia can usually be cured with vitamin D therapy within seven days.

Nerve dysfunction. – Just like the muscle cells, nerve cells are also activated by an inflow of calcium. If the necessary ignition voltage is lacking, the brain experiences the same problems as a computer with a poor power supply. If we are woken in the middle of the night, our intellectual capacities are initially quite limited. For patients with a severe vitamin D deficiency, they are like this permanently. A calcium deficiency in the brain resulting from a vitamin D deficiency impairs intellectual abilities. An undersupply of calcium causes disruptions in the nervous system, which in turn results in fitful sleep and insomnia, constant tiredness and exhaustion, impaired concentration, restlessness and internal anxiety.

This is also related to the fact that, when vascular muscles are not properly regulated by calcium ions, the dropping blood pressure is alternatively stabilized by the adrenaline system. However, this fire-fighting system stimulates the brain cells, which particularly causes problems at night. Once the deficiency is rectified, the symptoms dissipate promptly, usually within seven days.

Patients frequently complain about depression, sadness and melancholia. As the cause remains unknown if vitamin D levels are not measured, this depressive state is often incorrectly diagnosed as “endogenous depression”, for which, it is claimed, there are no external causes. In reality, many cases actually involve “secondary depression”, resulting from an ongoing lack of vitamin D. This is proven by the fact that it can be cured with vitamin D therapy. Depression can of course also have other causes which do not improve even with adequate vitamin D intake.

Orthostasis. – When you get up quickly after lying down, there is occasionally not enough blood pressure to properly supply all areas of the brain with blood, and everything goes black. The medical term for “upright position” is “orthostasis”. A vitamin D deficiency is probably the most significant cause of orthostatic problems, the so-called circulatory complaints. Rectifying the deficiency usually eases these complaints, as well as headaches occurring after getting up, headaches occurring after standing for a long time, nausea when under stress, ongoing head pressure, morning nausea, sensitivity to cold, pallor, and pins and needles in the arms and legs.

A vitamin D deficiency also causes vascular muscle dysfunction. Sphincters surround all blood-carrying tubes, much like a jet pilot’s pressurized suit. This prevents blood from being squeezed into the leg arteries and lacking in the brain as a result of radial acceleration when turning a curve, which would cause the pilot to suffer a life-threatening black-out. The sphincters’ activity is reduced when calcium is lacking. Getting up suddenly in the night can result in dizziness. A severe vitamin D deficiency can lead to a drop in blood pressure even in the day, with dizziness and impaired vision.

Pain and a feeling of pressure in the head are the products of counter-reactions. When the pressure sensors in the carotid arteries detect decreased blood pressure, an emergency reaction is produced: Adrenaline and similar hormones are suddenly released to stabilize blood pressure by activating the sphincters around the vessels. This adrenaline system turns on automatically, like a turbo. At higher doses, however, adrenaline and its relative, angiotensin, cause the vascular muscles in the head to cramp up, felt as a headache. This reflex often comes on so quickly that headaches begin straight after a black-out.

A serious vitamin D deficiency impairs continuous sphincter contraction due to the lack of calcium. The adrenaline system, which is actually only intended for emergency situations, must remain permanently active, which explains many patients' ongoing headaches.

Fitful sleep suffered by people with a vitamin D deficiency is the result of two mechanisms: the electrical instability of the nerve cells, and the unstable controlling of vascular muscles. Decreased muscle contraction during the night means the blood vessel sphincters are no longer stimulated by the adrenaline system, and blood pressure drops. However, the calcium system in people with vitamin D deficiency is not active enough. Blood accumulates in the arteries, which are too wide open, and blood pressure can reach critical values below 80 mmHg. During this night-time emergency, the adrenaline system switches on to prevent blood pressure from dropping further. The stimulative effect of the adrenaline on the brain results in disrupted sleep and causes the person to wake.

The often recommended milk and honey nightcap only

ever achieves limited, initial success, as the supply of calcium and sugar merely postpones the point at which the adrenaline system starts up. Sleep quality can only be permanently improved by rectifying the vitamin D deficiency.

Unfortunately, it is rarely possible to diagnose this correlation through blood pressure readings. If blood pressure is normal at night, we cannot know whether this figure is the result of intervention by the calcium system or the adrenaline system. Sweating, jerkiness and a high diastolic (second) blood pressure value may all be subtle indications of unwanted adrenaline system activity.

You sometimes hear people complain and say things such as "I don't like to play sport; it always makes me feel sick." Nausea occurring when playing sport is often another consequence of the adrenaline system suddenly kicking in. If someone who is not properly conditioned and is low in vitamin D starts running around, it is very likely they will be unable to keep going due to nausea and sometimes even vomiting.

Many patients complain of cold hands and feet. In some cases, their fingertips or entire hands go white, which is often the result of a cramp-like contraction of the blood vessel sphincters under the influence of adrenaline. This, too, can be improved through vitamin D treatment.

I have seen many patients with veins unsuitable for taking blood, but who, after months of vitamin D consumption, have ended up with healthy veins again. The sphincter cramps had obviously eased.

Orthostatic problems generally take longer to fix than other vitamin D deficiency symptoms. Once the deficiency has been rectified, it may take up to five weeks before any improvement is noticed. This delay is presumably the consequence of excessively weak sphincters, which need time to regain their strength.

Skeletal damage. – The fifth and final element of the MANOS concept is damage to the skeletal system. When people are vitamin-D deficient, their calcium intake and absorption is impaired, which is aggravated further by an incorrect diet. Overly acidic food (meat, fish, eggs, cheese, curd and cereals) increases calcium loss through the kidneys, while overly basic food (fruit and vegetables) minimizes this loss.

The blood must contain a consistently high concentration of calcium ions in order to maintain a healthy heart and brain function. However, calcium deficiencies resulting from vitamin D deficiency and increased losses through the kidneys can only be countered if the body draws on the calcium reserves in the bones. Bone mass is initially reduced at sites of low static importance: the cranial bone and breastbone are the first to be damaged by rickets. Once these calcium stores have been used up, the supporting bones also wear away, and bone density decreases. Osteoporosis develops steadily over time, increasing the risk of fractures. And it is not just among the elderly; younger people are increasingly also being affected by this.

The drop in bone mass is reversible in its early stages. Once it advances, however, trabeculae decompose, causing permanent damage which is initially asymptomatic. The size and shape of the vertebrae gradually change, which can lead to a change in spinal structure and chronic back pain. In some cases, the vertebrae even collapse, triggering excessive strain on the spinal disks. People suffering this sort of back pain often need more than a year of high vitamin D doses before the vertebrae can be restrengthened.

Vitamin D therapy does, however, work faster if the back pain is muscle-based.

Severe vitamin D deficiency impairs mineralization of the bones, which grow soft and may become deformed when strained. This is known as osteomalacia in adults, and rickets in children. The bending of softened bones causes the periosteum to tense, resulting in pain when under stress.

If foot and pelvic bones have become supple and soft due to osteomalacia, the groin area and feet will hurt when standing, though the pain will dissipate when lying down. These symptoms respond well to vitamin D therapy, but it takes months to achieve a noticeable improvement. Studies show that bone metabolism (AP enzyme) often takes over a year to normalize, so sufferers and therapists alike must be patient.

In severe cases of osteomalacia, the bones placed under strain when in a standing position are deformed, particularly the leg bones. This deformation is often permanent in children with rickets. To prevent lasting damage, a vitamin D deficiency must be diagnosed and rectified promptly before the bones become deformed.

If a patient is suffering from one or more of the MANOS symptoms, they may have an acute vitamin D deficiency. Their vitamin D levels must be checked, and any deficiency immediately rectified.

Complaints and illnesses can, of course, also have other causes, in which case they will not disappear after the treatment. In these instances, however, it is still advisable to maintain optimum vitamin D levels all year round as a preventive measure.

The calcium balance is not solely influenced by vitamin D levels; it is also affected by diet. Many of the so-called staple foods, such as refined sugar, candy, desserts, white flour products, oils and concentrated fats (butter, cream, margarine), meat and sausages, contain no or very little calcium. Even wholegrain products have low concentrations of calcium. The ratio of calcium to calories is inadequate. Furthermore, calcium is not readily available, since the small quantities of calcium which do exist are mostly bound to phytates and oxalates. Neither wholegrain nor white bread thus provides an adequate supply of calcium.

Excessively acidic food turns urine sour, which can be checked using a urine test strip. This means more calcium is lost through the kidneys, and the calcium balance is negative. To avoid this and reduce calcium loss, calorie requirements should preferably be met with highly basic foods, such as fruit, vegetables and potatoes.

Merely looking at the calcium content of food and recommending milk and dairy products will therefore not suffice. The extent to which the respective foods influence the acid/base equilibrium, and thus the calcium balance, is the crucial factor here. Although cheese and curd have high calcium concentrations, they lack base-forming substances, meaning lots of calcium is lost through the kidneys when vast quantities of highly acidic food are consumed. The balance is negative.

Vegetables, salads and low-calorie fruits have the highest concentrations of calcium and a high volume of excess base, though sweet fruits are also a good source of calcium. Potatoes are similarly basic, and should take preference over acidic cereal products such as bread, noodles or flour-based-dishes. The calcium concentration in potatoes is, however, kept within reasonable limits. Fruit and vegetables not only have high concentrations of calcium; they are also rich in vitamins, minerals and antioxidants.

Case studies

The names, exact ages and personal details in all case studies have been slightly modified to prevent identification.

Months of body aches

Mrs. Laguna (45) had been living in Germany for twenty years. She had increasingly been experiencing pain in all her joints, feet, hands and back over the last year. Everything hurt when she moved. The symptoms worsened at night and when resting. She soon found herself in agony when turning and rolling over at night. Finally, her entire body hurt, especially in the morning. Painkillers weren't working. She felt as if her whole body was swollen. The swellings could be seen around her eyes.

The standard laboratory tests and rheumatic factors revealed nothing, so she had to wait a further three months for an appointment with the rheumatologist. She was so exhausted, she could barely keep awake at work. "During this time, I would often tell myself I wouldn't be able to survive the day. I felt old, as if I were eighty, and thought 'why are you still even alive?'"

Her vitamin D levels were checked at a different practice, and she was told she was lacking in this vitamin. "I wondered, 'how can I be lacking in vitamins when I eat healthy?'" But she received no explanation. And the deficiency was unfortunately not addressed either.

The correct response would have been: People who avoid the sun cannot have normal vitamin D levels, and need to be treated with high doses of vitamin D.

Another check of her vitamin D levels at my practice showed a vitamin D value of 7.2 ng/ml, an extreme deficiency. Vitamin D therapy began. Within just one week, she was thrilled: “My pain subsided with each day that I took the vitamin D. Seven days later, all my pain had gone. I can hardly believe it, but I can cancel my appointment with the rheumatology.” And happy: “I can exercise again, and have already lost two kilos in a month.” She had also been suffering from a sun allergy for years. I encouraged her to try and sunbathe for ten minutes. One week later, she came back beaming, reporting that “I can tolerate the sun again – that is wonderful. I had always loved being in the sun as a child; I can now enjoy it again after all this time.”

When people have a vitamin D deficiency, their body can only absorb small quantities of calcium. The shortfall must be made up for using calcium from the bones. The body uses this precious bone mass sparingly. Bone degradation particularly slows down at night, meaning calcium levels drop during sleep. This makes sense, since the muscles are rarely needed at night. However, the low calcium levels result in muscle cramps, pain and poor circulation. Once vitamin D levels have been normalized, these night-time complaints disappear within a few days.

Dizziness caused by Menière's disease

Aged-care worker Mrs. Smith (48) had been suffering from dizziness for years, as if she were riding on a carousel, causing her to repeatedly miss weeks of work. Blood tests and MRIs revealed nothing. She was diagnosed with Menière's disease. The ENT specialist's attempts at treatment using drips, head injections and medication were fruitless.

In December, when she could barely walk from another bout of dizziness, her vitamin D levels were found to be 33.9 ng/ml. Despite this relatively good reading, she was first treated with 300,000 units, followed by weekly maintenance treatment with initially 20,000 units. A slight decline after one month was countered by increasing the dose to 40,000 units.

Five years have since passed, and she has not had another bout of dizziness. This shows that, when it comes to nervous system disorders, there is no harm in trying the therapy, even if vitamin D levels are between 30 and 40 ng/ml.

Everything hurts

Mrs. Pool (40), a factory worker, was depressed, with drooping shoulders and long face, when she came to see me: "I'm spent, I can't even raise my arms up anymore, everything hurts. I feel like I am laden down." She was also suffering muscle twitches and calf cramps. Upon further enquiry, I found out she was a smoker. She hadn't been in the sun over the last few months.

She was prescribed the vitamin D therapy in November, following a vitamin D reading of 10 ng/ml. Just a few days later, the muscle pain in her shoulders had disappeared, and the annoying muscle twitches had stopped. The patient had regained her strength.

This report contains symptoms from the M and A sections of the MANOS concept. The rapid improvement confirms the correlation with the vitamin D deficiency. Based on my experience, many factory workers suffer from this problem, as they work in closed rooms without any sun. Even their breaks are usually spent in closed rooms, and sunbathing at noon is often not possible. Many of them also smoke, thereby depleting their already modest vitamin D reserves. Frequent overtime on weekends similarly prevents them from getting the sun exposure they so urgently require.

Calf cramps

Mrs. Miller (37) had long been suffering from exhaustion, calf cramps and back pain. She had white lines on her fingernails, and was a smoker.

She underwent therapy to treat her vitamin D deficiency. Four days after her levels had been increased, all her complaints disappeared, though the fingernails take several months to regenerate themselves.

The symptoms of the M and A MANOS categories respond quickly to the vitamin D therapy.

Muscle twitches

By her own account, Mrs. Stone (44) was only getting two hours' sleep a night. She was suffering from night-time leg pain and muscle twitches.

After receiving vitamin D therapy, she reported that she was able to get restful, totally pain-free sleep from 9 pm to 6 am.

Medical textbooks barely mention night-time leg pain. The large-scale marketing of magnesium has obscured people's focus on simple, effective treatments using vitamin D.

Back pain

Mrs. Zelic (49) was experiencing incessant pain throughout her entire back, which slowed down the entire movement process. Her legs also hurt, and her calves cramped up at night. Her vitamin D levels were below the measurability threshold (less than 7 ng/ml). This was in mid-August. Her domestic lifestyle and the fact that her skin was covered by traditional clothing had prevented vitamin D from building up. The vitamin D therapy got rid of all her complaints.

The patient was suffering from migrant syndrome, characterized by a vitamin D deficiency and a number of resulting complaints. These are caused by the custom of avoiding the sun, which quickly proves to be detrimental in northern regions. Vitamin D deficiency is, however, also prevalent in the southern countries of origin, because even strong sunrays are useless if you are inside all the time and completely covered up.

Back and leg pain

Mrs. Bishop (77) was heavy footed when she came to see me in late April. She had back pain, and was also experiencing horrendous calf cramps every night. She was being bothered by pins and needles in the legs, and felt permanently listless.

Her vitamin D levels were at 9 ng/ml. She underwent vitamin D therapy, which instantly cured her fatigue and muscle problems. Her back and leg pain subsided after just a few weeks.

It never ceases to amaze me how even severe cases can be suddenly improved by rectifying a vitamin D deficiency.

Chronic fatigue

Mr. Covic (46) had been working at a factory for years. With his burly, somewhat overweight frame, he kept the boxes in the factory workshop moving, and ensured the production process ran smoothly. For months he had been coming home tired and falling asleep immediately. He had to avoid sitting down, because otherwise he would be overcome with fatigue. He felt healthy apart from this.

After undergoing the vitamin D therapy, his fatigue disappeared within a week. He was extremely satisfied with this treatment, as he was now able to get by on seven or eight hours' sleep.

Tiredness is certainly not an illness, and the cause should only be sought if it becomes a permanent state and is not due to lack of sleep. This means taking a vitamin D reading.

Lethargy

Mrs. Cook (46) was sent to me by her friend because she had been feeling so miserable in recent times. She complained of fatigue and lethargy. It was only upon further enquiry that she confirmed she also suffered from night-time muscle pain, muscle cramps in the legs, and back pain.

Everything subsided after the vitamin D therapy. Mrs. Cook was delighted to be able to have energy for her family again. In hindsight, she said: "I was really depressed."

Out of the M, A and N MANOS symptoms, depressiveness "N" is the most serious. People often say, "I can't sleep. If I could sleep, I would feel much better." What many people don't know, however, is that insomnia is a consequence of the vitamin D deficiency which must be rectified.

Fatigue

Childcare worker Mrs. Peers (36) reported that she was usually tired and jaded, and suffered from leg pain and calf cramps at night. Her fingernails displayed small white flecks. She had not taken a vacation in the sun for a long time, and never went to solariums. She had never been able to get any proper sun in the summer.

I prescribed her the vitamin D treatment. Three months later, we spoke by telephone, and she was thrilled to tell me that "I felt well again the very day I took the vitamin D capsules, full of energy and strength." The fatigue, which had lasted for months, had suddenly disappeared. Instead of having to go to bed at 8 pm like before, she was now able to stay up until 11 pm. Calf cramps and joint pain while sleeping were a thing of the past. She was able to get up every morning at 7 am feeling alert and well-rested.

The vitamin D therapy lifts people's moods and helps them overcome depressiveness. Many people really start to flourish.

Exhaustion

Mrs. Johnson (34) was completely exhausted. She had been suffering from ongoing fatigue and weariness for weeks. Her fingernails displayed white flecks, longitudinal grooves and brittle edges. She was plagued by calf cramps at night. She underwent vitamin D therapy, and one week later her fatigue and cramps had disappeared.

This medical report shows that muscles and the central nervous system are largely dependent on calcium supply. Calcium, in turn, is released by a feedback system with vitamin D, parathormone, calcitonin and calcitriol.

Vitamin D activation follows a day-night pattern, reaching its lowest point at night, which is why deficiency symptoms are more intense at night.

Neck pain

Ms. Dito (18) felt weak, and was suffering from neck pain and calf cramps. She smoked five cigarettes a day. Upon further enquiry, it was found that she never went in the sun because she felt unwell if she did so, and would get headaches and circulatory problems.

Her vitamin D levels in late November were 10 ng/ml, an extreme deficiency. Three days after this was normalized, her neck pain, calf cramps and fatigue disappeared.

Autonomic complaints are typical of a chronic vitamin D deficiency. When the skin is exposed to the sun, the blood vessels expand due to the warmth, intensifying circulatory problems and triggering headaches. Ms. Dito's complaints were able to be treated with vitamin D.

Limpness and weariness

Mr. Philipps (53) complained of endless weariness. For months he had been spending hours every day lying on the sofa, unable to pick himself up. Muscle twitches and calf cramps plagued him all day. His back pain had now become a permanent. He smoked a packet of cigarettes a day, which further aggravated the vitamin D deficiency.

His blood reading in September was 12 ng/ml, prompting vitamin D treatment. He returned in good spirits. The permanent fatigue and exhaustion had gone away, and even his wife admitted he was a completely different person. Muscle pain, muscle twitches and calf cramps had been gone for three days, as had the intense sweating, which had not been mentioned before. He was soon able to start working again.

Loss of appetite

Little Nadine (9) had for weeks been pale, tired, lackluster, and feeling dizzy when getting up. She had lost her appetite. She often ended up vomiting when she ate something. That was in mid-March.

She underwent vitamin D therapy in the children's dose. When I saw her again after a week, she came bounding into my room. All her complaints had gone away. Another week later, when we spoke by telephone, her mother confirmed everything was going swimmingly. Nadine was her old self again.

An acute vitamin D deficiency typically arises after a long period without sun, at the end of winter or in the spring. The amount of biologically effective sunshine we receive in our neck of the woods in winter is equal to zero. At the end of winter and during spring, most people's vitamin D levels have dropped to a pathologically low level. If they are still unable to sunbathe at noon in April and May, the deficiency persists.

Adynamia and debility

Mr. Baumann (61) was shockingly pale. He had already undergone multiple rounds of chemotherapy to treat his lung cancer. He felt feeble, utterly exhausted, fatigued and weak in all his limbs. His vitamin D level was 7 ng/ml. Once this was raised, he reported back five days later, delighted that he was able to climb the stairs again.

How can you activate your muscles when the calcium

needed to spark this activation is missing? Debilitation and a feeling of floppiness are the result.

It is tragic that cancer patients' general complaints are usually attributed to their underlying disease. This is a mistake. Cancer patients have a more urgent need for optimum vitamin D levels than other people.

No more morning blues after 15 years

Mrs. Childs (40) looked slightly aggrieved when she came slowly into my room, citing pain in the lower back, radiating out to her hips. During the consultation, she also confirmed she had been suffering from muscle cramps and fitful sleep. She had had a sun allergy for years, and smoked ten cigarettes a day.

She noticed an improvement after being treated with vitamin D. She cheerfully reported back, saying that "I'm always raring to go now when I wake up in the morning." For 15 years she had accepted she was just not a morning person. The first hour of the day had always been a struggle, because she had felt lackluster, tired and depressed. That was now suddenly a thing of the past, just like her sun allergy, which had for years been deemed as untreatable.

Allergic processes are normally suppressed by the vitamin D system, which is why patients are initially advised to still expose their skin to the sun despite their allergy. As vitamin D levels improve from the sunbathing, the skin itchiness usually also gradually subsides. This happens faster when sun allergy patients undergo vitamin D therapy before their first sunbathing session.

Emergency relief from exhaustion

Mrs. Georgina (51) came to my surgery for a prescription for flu medication. As she had been feeling so ill, she had hardly smoked a cigarette over the last few days. She was suffering from eyelid twitches, muscle twitches, muscle cramps and exhaustion. I prescribed vitamin D treatment, and advised her to give up smoking for good. A few days later, she returned to my room energized and full of life. "I feel ready to take on anything," she laughed. All her muscle complaints had disappeared, and she hadn't touched another cigarette.

Eyelid twitches, muscle twitches, muscle cramps and exhaustion are all symptoms of the M and A MANOS categories. They are very common, and respond quickly to vitamin D treatment.

Smokers are more likely to suffer these symptoms, as they are generally lower in vitamin D. Giving up smoking should thus be combined with vitamin D treatment. Based on my experience, this significantly decreases the probability of relapses.

The absent-minded apprentice

Apprentice Hans Meier (21) had for weeks been suffering from impaired concentration. He was forgetting his tasks at work, and mixing up colors and components.

In August, his vitamin D level was just 17 ng/ml. Despite spending time outdoors, his smoking habit had obviously contributed to the low reading. His concentration problems dissipated once his vitamin D was increased.

This report shows the significant impact vitamin D has on retention and intellectual capacity.

Migraines

Mrs. Holmes (36) often came to see me for her migraines. She also suffered from fatigue and back pain. Her muscles often cramped up and twitched. Her circulation was so impaired she was barely in a fit state.

At the end of April, her vitamin D level was 13 ng/ml. I started her on vitamin D treatment. She felt better after a few weeks of medium doses of vitamin D. Her circulatory complaints had disappeared, and her muscles had also stopped twitching. Even the back pain, which had plagued her for months, had subsided. She was experiencing one tenth of the migraines she used to have.

Autonomic disorders, such as chronic headaches and migraines, are typical of a chronic vitamin D deficiency. The treatment is effective, simple and safe.

Dizziness

Mr. Lehmann (63) had for months been plagued by nighttime calf cramps and pins and needles in the legs. A persistent dizziness would often come over him when he stood up. He was initially diagnosed as having circulatory problems, though magnesium tablets did not help much.

In late April, his vitamin D level was found to be 15 ng/ml. I started him on vitamin D treatment, and one week later his calf cramps and all circulatory problems had disappeared.

Attention deficit disorder and hyperactivity

Alex (8) was always fidgety and wired up; his hyperactivity was a pain in the neck for his parents and siblings. He could never fall asleep before midnight. His vitamin D level was 22 ng/ml. Once it was increased, he was able to go to sleep at a more normal time of 9 pm.

Trembling

Ms. Anders (19), a salesperson by profession, was seeking help after weeks of intense fatigue. On her days off, she would spend hours sleeping, and even then was unable to pick herself up. A trembling in her arms had been getting worse and worse, and had often seen her spill powdered substances at work. Plagued by muscle twitches in her calves, thighs, arms and face, she was also mentally troubled.

A vitamin D reading in October showed a severe deficiency (16 ng/ml). She started vitamin D therapy, which got rid of most of her symptoms. The annoying muscle twitches and day-time fatigue largely disappeared. Her sleep was also much less fitful than before. She noticed that her hands, which had otherwise always been cold and bluish, were now pleasantly warm. Months later she reported that her fingernails were no longer breaking.

An activated adrenaline system triggers muscle tremors. By normalizing the vitamin D system, which impacts on circulation, the adrenaline system's activity can be reduced, and the associated complaints cured.

Dizziness and headaches

Mrs. George (35) had been suffering from serious circulation problems. Her blood pressure would drop sharply as soon as she stood up. Her vision was impaired, dizziness would force her to the ground; her blood pressure was below 100 mmHg. She had been plagued by headaches for weeks. Sometimes her condition was so bad that I had to make a house call to give her an injection so she could get back on her feet. When all attempts failed, we decided to administer cortisone. It only helped insofar as it was being injected. The patient consulted a series of other doctors and alternative practitioners, to no avail.

In June 2006, I called the patient and suggested doing a blood test. I was shocked to find a total lack of vitamin D (less than 7 ng/ml). I started her on vitamin D treatment. A few weeks later, the dizziness, which had persistently plagued her, had completely stopped. Her migraines had also subsided, as had the thigh muscle twitches and daytime fatigue. She also attributed her reduction in cold sores to the vitamin treatment. She noticed that sun exposure no longer caused her headaches. This improvement confirms the cause as being a vitamin D deficiency. The patient has not suffered any such crises in subsequent years.

Persistently low blood pressure is not always the result of a cortisone deficiency; it can also be due to a vitamin D deficiency. Both steroid hormones are necessary for proper blood pressure. Unlike cortisone, there are no risks associated with vitamin D treatment.

This medical report shows that the central nervous system and vascular muscles are largely dependent on a sufficient supply of calcium. Serious vitamin D deficiency can result in severe complaints caused by an impaired autonomic nervous system.

Depression

Mrs. Opaker (63) trudged into my consultation room. She was suffering from headaches, joint pain, back pain and exhaustion. Her companions reported that insomnia, pain and unrest meant nights were extremely draining. Treatment had allegedly been performed based on the diagnoses of "fibromyalgia, somatic depression and painkiller abuse", but did not provide relief. The patient spent all her time at home, avoiding the sun due to constant headaches.

Laboratory tests in September confirmed a total lack of vitamin D (less than 7 ng/ml). As expected, bone metabolism (AP – alkaline phosphatase) was also highly active. She was prescribed vitamin D treatment, and all symptoms subsided after two weeks.

Sleep disorders

Mrs. Adler (72) had for weeks been complaining of fitful sleep, calf cramps and nightmares. Her husband said she would constantly toss and turn in bed at night. Regular magnesium intake had not brought any significant improvement.

She underwent vitamin D therapy. A few days later, she said the calf cramps had disappeared and she was able to sleep peacefully again.

The fact that these symptoms usually occur at night can be explained by the drop in active vitamin D during sleep. There is a circadian rhythm (24-hour rhythm) at work here, which drops to its lowest point at night, causing the symptoms of acute vitamin D deficiency, particularly at night.

Hallucinations: Hearing voices

Mrs. Demir (31) was exhausted and distraught, and came to her consultation with tears streaming down her face. She complained of pain, fear and exhaustion. For months she had been working the early shift at a factory, from 6am to 2pm. It was only upon further enquiry that she mentioned she was plagued by calf cramps every night. Some muscles would often hurt and twitch. She was also experiencing pain in her lower back. She constantly felt dizzy, and had blackouts when she stood up suddenly. She smoked a pack of cigarettes a day.

Upon my questioning, she confirmed that she had noticed "her thoughts becoming louder". She could hear all of them as a whispering voice. She hadn't told anyone about this, because she feared she would be labeled as "crazy". Her vitamin D level was only 12 ng/ml. Two days after starting vitamin D treatment, she returned radiant. The calf cramps and muscle pain in her legs had gone. She had not felt any pins and needles in her hands. She was able to sleep normally again, and was particularly grateful for this. But the most important thing for this patient was that the depressive moods and whispering voices had disappeared, as had the exhaustion and anxiety. "It's been months since I have had such joie de vivre."

"Autonomic complaints" are typical of a chronic vitamin D deficiency. "Hearing whispering voices" is another symptom. Observant doctors also encounter this phenomenon in patients low in calcium. They often refrain from mentioning this symptom due to their fear of being treated as mentally deranged. This is usually prematurely diagnosed as a schizoid disease (psychosis, schizophrenia). In doing so, people often forget that psychoses can also have other causes, and that, in such cases, it is advisable to check vitamin D levels and quickly rectify the deficiency instead of routinely prescribing antipsychotics.

Raynaud's circulatory disorders

Mr. Dollier (78) had for weeks been noticing increasing pain in all his muscles. Upon further questioning, he also confirmed he suffered from calf cramps. He similarly had problems with circulation in his fingers; sometimes they were numb, as if they had died. He felt extremely weary and constantly exhausted.

The standard laboratory readings did not reveal anything, except that his vitamin D was 16 ng/ml (in April). After rectifying the deficiency, all his complaints disappeared. He was full of energy and pain-free once more. Even his fingers stayed warm.

In this case, the symptoms in the Muscles, Adynamia and Orthostasis MANOS categories include impaired finger circulation, also known as Raynaud's disease. The complaints resulting from the vascular spasms improved as vitamin D increased. Even this baffling disease is thus curable, insofar as it is caused by a vitamin D deficiency.

Morning vomiting

Mr. Fitzgerald (67) had for months been suffering gag reflex and vomiting every morning. Almost every day, he would have to stop on the way to work to vomit on the side of the street. He also complained of a distinct, ongoing feeling of weakness. His movements had become impaired due to back pain and pins and needles in the legs. All conceivable types of tests had been performed, countless laboratory readings calculated, and all nausea and upset stomach medication tried. But to no avail; there had been no improvement.

In mid-April, his vitamin D level was just 13 ng/ml. After undergoing vitamin D treatment, his vomiting and gag reflex had disappeared, as had his circulatory complaints and exhaustion.

Almost every night, Ina and Tina (5 and 3) would wake up and complain of pain in the legs, especially the knees, calves and feet. Their mother had to keep gently massaging their feet and toes. As there did not appear to be any other problems, she thought it was just a quirk particular to the two girls.

The children were given 5,000 units of vitamin D every day for a week. At the follow-up, the mother reported that the children were sleeping well again, with no more pain.

Parents often find that their young children complain of leg pain during the night. When they check their legs by hand, they are found to be sensitive to pressure. They look for signs of injury, but there are none. The pain appears when the child is in the correct posture. The fact that they wake up at night also indicates a physical cause, rather than a mental one.

Most parents and doctors are perplexed, so the child is taken to an orthopedic specialist, who cannot find anything beyond the pseudo-diagnosis of "growth pain". Even an X-ray shows nothing. If the vitamin D deficiency goes undetected as the cause, the complaints persist. They are often expected to "go away on their own", which only happens if the child sunbathes in UVB radiation.

An acute vitamin D deficiency typically appears towards the end of spring, when six months have passed since vitamin D was last formed through sun exposure.

This case study shows that a growing child's muscles and skeleton are largely dependent on good calcium intake and vitamin D level. The so-called growth pains are typical of a chronic vitamin D deficiency. Vitamin D therapy is simple and safe. Most complaints disappear within a week when treated with high doses of vitamin D.

Sun allergy

Diana and Jonas (10 and 12) were brought in to see me by their mother because of an annual sun allergy. "It's our fifth year going to the seaside, and the two of them always get a fierce sun allergy. What can we do about this? We've tried everything; allergy tablets and all kinds of sun creams, but nothing has helped."

I recommended taking 2,000 units of vitamin D a day for the three weeks leading up to their departure. Upon their return, I was told none of the sun allergy symptoms had appeared.

Sun allergies can be treated by normalizing vitamin D levels. On the other hand, those who try to counter them using sun cream will end up in a vicious circle, as sun cream actually prevents vitamin D from forming. Unfortunately, a lot of money is made out of this misleading illusion. The cosmetics industry also contributes to this misinformation, earning hefty profits from sunscreens, and concealing these side effects.

Allergy

Mr. Wilkins (52) complained of annual pollen allergies which were once again troubling him. He also had cross sensitivity to apples and nuts, which caused an instant itchiness in the mouth. Upon further questioning, he mentioned he suffered from calf cramps at night and muscle twitches in the day. He regarded back pain and ongoing exhaustion as inevitable. His fingernails were dull and ribbed.

His vitamin D level in May was just 9 ng/ml. This was normalized. By the time he came for his follow-up, his muscle twitches and calf cramps had disappeared. At subsequent appointments, the patient reported he was no longer suffering back pain. The circulatory complaints, which had previously appeared every time he straightened up, had also ceased. Finally, he mentioned he was able to eat apples again without noticing any itchiness in the mouth.

Prescribing calcium alone will only improve acute allergic symptoms for a few hours. They will not be permanently cured unless the vitamin D deficiency is rectified.

Asthma and susceptibility to infection

Anna (10) had been suffering from asthmatic bronchitis since the age of seven. The obstructive bronchitis was treated by the lung specialist as suspected incipient asthma. Every time she caught a cold, Tina felt breathless; she coughed incessantly day and night, and a whistling noise could be heard every time she breathed in.

She took a vitamin D dose of 1,000 units a day over an

extended period of time. The following year, when she was eight, she caught colds which also caused noticeable breathlessness. By increasing her vitamin D intake, however, she was able to withstand infections and asthma all year round by the ages of nine and ten.

Many parents wonder what they can do to protect their children from asthma and infectious diseases. The immune system is highly dependent on vitamin D, which is why people primarily suffer from asthma and infections in winter and spring, when vitamin D levels are at their lowest. Ten-year-olds undergoing permanent treatment should take at least 2,000 units a day.

Nervous breakdown

Mr. Holland (44) had a lot on his plate. He worked from 6am to 4pm, after which he would go and build his house. He had stopped taking holidays in order to keep building. He had come for a consultation because he felt completely spent: "I think I'm having a nervous breakdown!" His muscles were sore. He would fall asleep instantly every evening at 8pm, and felt nauseous when he got up in the morning. He had a subliminal anxiety, was often gripped by internal unrest, and sometimes found himself crying.

I prescribed vitamin D. Three days later, all his symptoms had disappeared. He had no more pain in his muscles, and was able to work on his house until midnight. His mood had changed too; he was cheerful instead of depressed.

Back pain and weakness

Mr. Oeztuerk (25) was suffering from ongoing pain and a feeling of weakness. He had long been trying to endure the back pain so as not to lose his job. His fingernails displayed numerous white flecks. He had been plagued by night-time muscle cramps for some time. The pain in his back was worse when he spent a long time standing, and spread as far as both groin areas. He was a smoker.

The patient underwent vitamin D treatment. One week later, his cramps and weariness had disappeared, and his back pain had significantly subsided.

This case shows an unusually rapid response to vitamin D intake. It was presumably the muscle dysfunction which contributed to the intense malaise.

Brittle fingernails

Mrs. Jansen (47) had been unhappy with her fingernails for ten years; they would snap, chip or split in two. She underwent vitamin D treatment. Two to three months later, her fingernails were back to normal.

Fingernail strength is largely dependent on good calcium intake. The two to three-month time frame is equivalent to the time needed for fingernails to regenerate themselves.

Myocardial insufficiency

Mr. Clearwater (83) was discharged from hospital with no hope of a cure, and left to die at home. Although he was taking ten different types of heart medication, his heart was giving way. Water had built up in his legs. Despite all treatment, they had remained edematous. His vitamin D level was below the measurability threshold, i.e. less than 7 ng/ml.

He underwent vitamin D therapy and experienced a noticeable improvement. After a few weeks, he was walking in the street, and some time later he was able to make it through the entire village and around the church. Five years later, he is still enjoying life.

This report shows that cardiac muscles are also highly dependent on a good supply of calcium. Calcium is systematically released by a mechanism involving vitamin D, parathormone, calcitonin and calcitriol. Heart failure is a typical symptom of a long-time vitamin D deficiency. It is not due to age in itself, but rather due to the fact that many old people do not get enough sun.

Tinnitus

Mrs. Conolly (54) had noticed an increasing noise in both ears within the space of a few days. She had spent an entire year seeing many different doctors, as well as an ENT university hospital, but to no avail.

It was not until the patient took a high dose of vitamin D over four days that she noticed an improvement. The noise in her ears got better each day. Within three weeks, she was largely symptom-free. She kept taking vitamin D to maintain a good level. She did not experience any relapses in a follow-up period of five years.

There is evidently a type of tinnitus which is dependent on vitamin D. There is no reason not to treat such symptoms as those of a vitamin D deficiency.

Enteritis

Mr. Walter (60) came to see me because his inflammatory bowel disease with bloody stools had not improved under cortisone treatment. He avoided sunshine, as this made him feel unwell and break out into a sweat. He even avoided sunlight when on holidays. He held a responsible position with a heavy workload.

Two weeks after the vitamin D therapy, he reported he had stopped experiencing bloody diarrhea. Every cortisone treatment should be coupled with vitamin D intake. This indication is often neglected, because it is incorrectly assumed the patient's vitamin D level is adequate. Reality shows, however, that it is actually completely the opposite. As a biochemical relative of cortisone, vitamin D also controls the immune system.

Colitis with Raynaud's disease

I made house calls to see Mrs. Green (79), as she was not strong enough to leave her home. She was suffering from unexplained heart failure. She had pain and pins and needles in her legs. Inflamed bowels with bloody diarrhea had become serious. The patient was in poor health. Her hands were always blue and ice cold. The hospital had kept recommending cortisone tablets and anti-inflammatory enemas to combat unspecified colitis, but there was no improvement.

Her vitamin D level in May was 15 ng/ml. I started her on vitamin D treatment, and her bloody diarrhea stopped within just a few days. The patient's condition improved rapidly. After a year without relapse, it was clear that her colitis had been cured. Her veins, whose cramps had always made it difficult to take blood, were clearly visible again on both forearms. Her calves, which had been thin and hard, were now soft and supple. Her once ice-cold fingers now had proper circulation again. Her ability to work under pressure in everyday life had also improved. Her hemoglobin (Hb) values had risen from 7.8 to 13 g/l.

For the cortisone treatment alone, it is a doctor's duty to reduce the harmfulness of cortisone by normalizing vitamin D levels, otherwise bone mass will be lost.

Heartburn

Mr. Bernstein (43) suffered heartburn whenever he ate brown bread. For years, he had been experiencing this pain behind his breastbone and in his upper abdomen, which also occurred after eating other foods.

He underwent vitamin D treatment for general health purposes. Three months later, as part of another appointment, he reported his heartburn had disappeared as soon as he had started the vitamin D therapy. He was able to eat brown bread again whenever he wanted. Pain, which had been recurring for years, had stopped.

The smooth muscles in the stomach and intestine, which are controlled by the autonomic nervous system, are heavily dependent on good vitamin D level. As evidenced by this case study, a vitamin D deficiency can obviously lead to heartburn.

Multiple sclerosis and neuropathic pain

Dr. Wagner (53), a specialist in internal medicine, had suffered from multiple sclerosis for eleven years. He also experienced constant fatigue, muscle twitches and neuropathic pain.

After doing some research on the Internet, he decided to check his vitamin D levels. Following high doses of vitamin D and regular visits to the solarium, his level was recorded at 72 ng/ml. From then on, he took a maintenance dose.

The fatigue and night-time muscle twitches have not recurred since. The neuropathic pain has improved and only occurs very rarely. We are yet to see the extent to which the progression of multiple sclerosis can be slowed down. A benefit is already apparent. We also know that vitamin D deficiency significantly increases the risk of developing multiple sclerosis.

His own successes prompted the doctor to check his own patients' vitamin D levels. The results were alarming: Around 95 percent had low readings below 30 ng/ml. The one exception was a pensioner, with a reading of 42 ng/ml. He had been able to take seven holidays to the sunny Mediterranean in the course of one year. A solarium-goer also recorded a reading of 40 ng/ml.

All of the doctor's deficient patients underwent vitamin D therapy based on the principles described in this book. Symptoms disappeared in most cases.

Conclusion

These case studies show how important it is to check vitamin D levels, and raise these immediately if a deficiency is detected.

If checked regularly, vitamin D deficiency would be one of the most common pathological laboratory finding. This should become a routine procedure, in light of the serious effects it can have.

It would be advisable for all health funds to reimburse expenses for the vitamin D test in suspect cases. This would save on the high costs resulting from medical examinations and treatments, inability to work, and stays at health resorts, not to mention the vast sequelae caused by incorrect prescriptions.

Normal, natural, optimum vitamin D levels

Laboratory readings of healthy people are considered normal. But health is a subjective matter. Excluding malaise and autonomic complaints such as muscle twitches, muscle pain, a high need for sleep, headaches and circulatory complaints, many vitamin D-deficient patients are classified as healthy, and low average readings deemed normal, even though that is not correct. Degenerative diseases similarly progress unnoticed for years, during which time the persons affected are mistakenly classed among the healthy.

So we should not ask what is normal in a population characterized by illness. We must instead strive for the values needed to maintain health and energy levels even in old age. In other words, it is the *optimum*, not the average, and therefore statistically *normal*, vitamin D level which we should be focusing on as the target value.

The average annual vitamin D level in Germany is 16 ng/ml. The average in winter is between 8 and 12 ng/ml, and in summer around 24 ng/ml. Readings below 20 ng/ml are usually accompanied by autonomic complaints, such as fatigue, weariness, fitful sleep, leg pain and muscle twitches.

Leading a natural lifestyle does not necessarily mean vitamin D levels will be optimum. Even those who are able to take advantage of every opportunity to sunbathe at noon will only reach a good vitamin D level of over 40 ng/ml after 15 to 30 sunny days in spring.

No vitamin D can be built up in northern countries during the winter months from October to March, as the sun's low position means UVB radiation in the atmosphere is filtered out and does not reach the earth's surface. Without UVB sunlight on the skin, vitamin D levels drop by around 20 percent a month, unless they are boosted through artificial UVB radiation or medications. Food does not have any major influence here.

The vitamin D levels achieved through natural lifestyles are thus highly dependent on the season and weather.

Sunseekers do not necessarily achieve optimum vitamin D levels either, even in summer, as UVB radiation is blocked out by sunscreen, preventing vitamin D from forming. Many people don't sun themselves at midday when the sun is at its highest and UVB radiation is at its maximum, but rather at other times when only very little vitamin D can be formed.

An ideal vitamin D intake all year round can only be achieved in the tropics, outer tropics and in Mediterranean countries (Greece, southern Spain and southern Italy in Europe, southern states in the U.S.), provided the entire body is exposed to at least a brief amount of sun at midday on every sunny day.

On the other hand, it is impossible to form vitamin D for five to six months during the winter in England and Scotland or in Canada, due to the sun's low position.

Natives in equatorial countries usually achieve vitamin D levels of between 30 and 90 ng/ml, which is deemed natural. But even in the event of excessive sun exposure, there is no risk of vitamin D levels rising above 100 ng/ml. Overdosing is not possible using natural methods.

Satisfactory calcium intake can be expected if vitamin D

levels are over 30 ng/ml, but the best results for preventing osteoporosis in old age are only achieved if they remain over 40 ng/ml all year round. Vitamin D levels over 55 ng/ml must be aimed for in order to ensure the best protection against cancer.

Definitions:

1. *Acute vitamin D deficiency.* The term acute (Latin for sharp) in this case relates to the possibility of rapid improvement. All of the syndrome's complaints and symptoms disappear within a month of achieving optimum vitamin D levels.
2. *Chronic vitamin D deficiency.* The consequences of a long-time deficiency may be irreparable, though vitamin D treatment can bring an improvement, even after one year.

Vitamin D

1 µg = 40 International Units (IU)

Vitamin D level in the blood

1 ng/ml = 1 µg/l = 2.5 nmol/l

Conversion factors for the quantity and concentration of vitamin D in the blood (25-hydroxycholecalciferol, 25-OH-D_3).

Toxic effect	over 300 ng/ml
Risk of excessively high calcium	over 150 ng/ml
Recommended upper limit in the blood	100 ng/ml
Level with regular sunbathing	50 to 90 ng/ml
Optimal (minimum risk of illness)	50 to 90 ng/ml
Good (low susceptibility to illness)	over 40 ng/ml
Satisfactory (good calcium intake)	over 30 ng/ml
Deficiency (risk of osteoporosis in old age)	under 30 ng/ml
Serious deficiency (high osteoporosis risk, autonomic nervous system disorder)	under 20 ng/ml
Extreme deficiency (osteomalacia, rickets)	under 12 ng/ml

Vitamin D levels in the blood's serum (25-OH-D_3).

It is believed that the best way to protect against degenerative disorders and infectious diseases is to ensure vitamin D levels remain above 40 ng/ml. Values below this result in a greater susceptibility to illness, and poorer overall health (www.grassrootshealth.org).

Those who use every sunny day to expose their entire body to a moderate amount of sun at midday will reach values between 50 and 90 ng/ml by the end of summer. It is not possible to overdose on vitamin D when sunbathing, because high vitamin D levels also trigger a reverse reaction which brings them back down, thus guaranteeing a natural equilibrium at a high level.

Things get critical in winter. Even those who start fall with high vitamin D levels will drop below 30 ng/ml by the end of the winter if they do not take a supplement or get exposure to UVB radiation. Most are well below this limit.

Calculating vitamin D levels

Despite vitamin D deficiency being widespread, patients' blood levels are rarely tested. In some cases, the test is not even performed when deficiency symptoms are present. Most doctors do not yet realize that a vitamin D deficiency is the cause of many illnesses. The latest research findings have so far only been taken onboard by very few physicians. Pharmaceutical companies have no reason to change this situation, because vitamin D is cheap and does not generate much profit.

Given the serious consequences of a vitamin D deficiency, patients are advised to take the initiative if they suspect they are suffering from one. These suspicions are often confirmed by a laboratory test.

Calculating the vitamin D level in blood (25-hydroxycholecalciferol) is relatively expensive. Laboratories charge around 70 $ for it. In normal cases, there is no need to test the concentration of active vitamin D (1,25- hydroxycholecalciferol) on top of this.

- *25-hydroxycholecalciferol* (25-OH-D) also known as *calcidiol*, is the inactive storage form of vitamin D. This book always refers to this 25-vitamin D value, because only it can provide information on how well stocked the vitamin D stores are. The 25-vitamin D level is stable during the day, though sunbathing and medication can raise it in the hours which follow. Without vitamin D supplements or skin exposure to UVB radiation, the 25-vitamin D level drops 10 to 30 percent per month (around 20 percent on average).

- *1,25-hydroxycolecalciferol* (1,25-$(OH)_2$–D_3), also known as *calcitriol*, is the active form of vitamin D, as this compound activates the vitamin D receptors in the cell nuclei. The active form is measured in pg/ml (picogram: 10^{-12} g) and the storage form in ng/ml (nanogram: 10^{-9} g). The blood level of active vitamin D is thus only one thousandth of the inactive form. Conversion of the stored 25-vitamin D to the active 1,25-vitamin D varies greatly, and is constantly adjusted as necessary. This value increases when muscles are active, which is why 1,25-vitamin D concentration in the blood fluctuates considerably. There is generally no need to calculate the level of active vitamin D. The critical factor is how well stocked the vitamin D stores are.

Given the serious consequences of a vitamin D deficiency, this is money well spent for patients. Laboratory costs are negligible in this respect. Alternatively, the levels can also be estimated if intake is clearly low.

Calculation of vitamin D levels as the basis for further treatment

If a vitamin D deficiency is suspected, it is a good idea to perform a laboratory test, which clarifies the severity of the deficiency. The right dose for the vitamin D treatment can then be determined. Having optimum vitamin D levels is essential for restoring and maintaining health. Around eighty percent of our patients suffering from an *acute vitamin D deficiency* notice some sort of improvement, and often even experience a complete recovery.

The vitamin D test is also recommended for treating or preventing chronic degenerative diseases, many of which are aggravated by a vitamin D deficiency. This has been proven for rickets and osteomalacia (bone softening and deformation), osteoporosis, cancers, reduced intellectual capacity, tuberculosis, susceptibility to infections, weakened immunity, and autoimmune diseases.

Though pale, sallow skin is an indication of vitamin D deficiency, it has long been known that tanned skin is not proof of satisfactory or optimum vitamin D levels, since tanning is also stimulated by UVA radiation (instant pigmentation, as opposed to slow, ongoing tanning from UVB radiation). A certain amount of tanning can be achieved in just one single sunbathing session, whereas vitamin D levels usually be raised by about 2 ng/ml, even if the entire body is exposed to intense UVB radiation.

And it is often only the skin on the face, hands and forearms which become tanned, while the rest remains pale, because sunlight has not reached the entire body. Very little vitamin D is thus gained. Pale skin on the body is indicative of a deficiency, even if the face is tanned.

When the sun's position is low and the air hazy, a noticeable tan can be achieved from UVA radiation after a few sunbathing sessions, even though hardly any vitamin D-promoting UVB radiation has reached the earth's surface. Here, once again, the tanned skin is a false indictor of good vitamin D level.

Sunscreens prevent vitamin D from forming, as they block UVB radiation. Redness is delayed, meaning people end up spending too long in the sun. UVA radiation, however, passes through a lot of the sunscreen chemicals, stimulating skin pigmentation. Those who use sun cream every time they sunbathe may well get a tan, but will still suffer a vitamin D deficiency.

A lack of sunshine is easy to pick in fair-skinned people. This is not the case for southerners due to their general skin pigmentation. In addition, people with darker skin (skin types 4 to 6) need more UVB radiation than those with pale skin to build up the same amount of vitamin D. People with very dark (black) skin need ten times more UVB radiation than white Europeans. As there is no sunbathing culture in their countries of origin, since the sun shines intensely there all year round, they quickly develop a severe vitamin D deficiency (in northern countries) due to their avoidance of the sun and indifference towards sunbathing. Vitamin D tests should confirm this deficiency.

Visual diagnoses can also be deceptive for pale-skinned people if the skin's tan fades faster than the vitamin D level drops. So not everyone who looks pale in winter is necessarily vitamin D-deficient. Given all these uncertainties surrounding visual diagnoses, doctors should become more aware of vitamin D, and talk to patients about their lifestyles. How often have they sunbathed in recent times? At what time of the day? Did they expose their whole body? With or without sunscreen? Where did they spend their last vacation? Do they regularly go to a solarium and do they actually use a UVB emitter? Do they take vitamin D supplements? If so, in what dose? Do they bear sunlight without complications? The often negative responses to these questions confirm that a vitamin D test is needed.

Older people frequently have a reduced ability to form vitamin D, meaning that, after sunbathing, their vitamin D level rises less than that of a younger.

Tobacco consumption, excess weight and obesity, living in enclosed spaces, living in big cities (haze from air pollutants reduces the intensity of UVB radiation), working in factories or offices, frequent night shifts (meaning even sunny days are slept through), not going outdoors at noon and exposing skin to the sun, using sun cream when sunbathing, and taking medication which disturbs the vitamin D metabolism (antiepileptics such as *Phenytoin* or *Carbamazepine*) are all reasonable grounds for suspecting a deficiency.

Professor Michael Holick recommends a test for initial diagnosis: Pressing on a patient's breastbone with the thumb triggers pain if mild or full-blown osteomalacia is present. The Holick test thus only allows us to infer whether the periosteum has swelled over a longer period of time due to a vitamin D deficiency. But it should never come to this critical state. If, on the other hand, the Holick test does not produce any pain, this is by no means proof of a good vitamin D level. The patient could still be suffering a severe deficiency.

Normal calcium levels should not prevent vitamin D levels from being checked

Many people think that checking calcium levels will suffice. As these are usually normal, they assume they are getting enough calcium. But they are mistaken. Their bodies are forced to draw on the calcium reserves in the bones to ensure nerves and muscles function correctly, including the myocardium. Excessively low calcium levels would result in a collapse with convulsions.

The calcium level in the blood is thus not a reliable indicator of the overall calcium balance. Calcium levels can be normal even if significant amounts of calcium are lost through the kidneys and calcium intake via the intestine is poor. The body can be suffering from an extreme calcium deficiency, and be in calcium-saving mode, while blood levels will still be showing as normal. Despite the normal calcium readings, the symptoms and complaints of an acute vitamin D deficiency then start to appear, and chronic deficiency-based diseases develop over time.

General statements on calcium absorption and utilization can only be made if vitamin D levels are included. This value alone indicates whether or not vitamin D treatment is needed.

Calcium levels of 2.1 or 2.2 mmol/l in the lower normal region are, however, suggestive of a serious vitamin D deficiency.

The AP value as a review and monitoring instrument

There is good reason to suspect bone deterioration if alkaline phosphatase (AP) values are well over 100 U/l (units per liter) when liver values are normal. High readings of over 120 U/l sometimes indicate advanced osteoporosis. AP values usually drop to around 50 to 80 U/l after one or two years of vitamin D treatment.

As AP values are cheap to test, and are checked often, it

is worth looking for high readings in the patient record, as these may indicate a past vitamin D deficiency. Raised AP values mean vitamin D levels should also be checked.

It is also a good idea to regularly test AP levels to monitor osteoporosis patients, though people with low body weights often have normal AP values even if they are extremely vitamin D-deficient. It is essential to check their vitamin D levels.

Reference values of AP should be viewed with caution. The limit value for adults has been set at 100 U/l, while it is 140 U/l for the elderly. But bone degeneration is already occurring at these levels, aided by the usually concomitant vitamin D deficiency. In children, AP values up to 500, or indeed even up to 700 U/l, are classified as "normal for their age", even though vitamin D treatment can halve these high readings in a short space of time.

Only AP values achieved after an extended period of good vitamin D levels should be deemed safe and normal. For adults, this is usually in the region of between 50 and 80 U/l.

Vitamin D treatment

Focusing on stores rather than daily requirements

Vitamin D stores in deficient patients are empty, and need to be replenished. This is why the treatment is broken down into:

1. *The initial treatment.* Serves to replenish stores and quickly reach an optimum vitamin D level. The required dose is taken once within a few days. Body weight and the difference between the target value and actual 25-vitamin D level are the definitive factors.
2. *Ongoing treatment.* Serves to balance out daily losses and maintain a good level of vitamin D, based on daily or weekly requirements.

Many people make the mistake of not undergoing the initial treatment, thereby failing to reach an optimum vitamin D level in the first week and bring about a speedy recovery.

The second common mistake is to prescribe an inadequate maintenance dose for the ongoing treatment. The standard baby doses of 400 or 800 units will do nothing. This dose for infants with a body weight of three kilograms was purely aimed at preventing rickets. Adults' requirements are much greater.

The key is to ensure that optimum vitamin D levels are achieved right at the start, and then maintained. A sufficient stock of vitamin D must be built up and guaranteed so that the body can draw on this and perform its vitamin D tasks.

Legal information: The following recommended doses are based on well-founded knowledge from specialist literature and years of practical clinical experience gained at an expert level. However, every doctor and therapist is obliged to keep themselves up to date on vitamin D treatment developments, to perform detailed examinations for each case and adapt the treatment according to the individual situation.

If there is a suspected deficiency, it is advisable to check the patient's vitamin D levels (experts can omit the test for patients who have lacked vitamin D intake for a long period of time). Based on this finding, the doctor will assess whether or not vitamin D treatment is needed, calculating a dose for the initial treatment and a daily dose for the ongoing treatment.

The therapy is recommended for blood levels below 30 ng/ml. If symptoms and illnesses caused by a vitamin D deficiency are noted, these must be cured. The same applies when reducing the risk of degenerative diseases aggravated by vitamin D deficiency. There is no reason not to treat vitamin D deficiency with the exception of an active sarcoidosis.

Vitamin D levels of over 40 ng/ml are desirable for osteoporosis patients in order to prevent bone degeneration. A permanent target value above 50 ng/ml is advisable to protect against cancer.

Vitamin D levels should be below 100 – 150 ng/ml. People who expose their bodies to intense UVB radiation on a daily basis, e.g. pool attendants in summer and natives of tropical regions, remain below 100 ng/ml.

A vitamin D level of up to 150 ng/ml appears not to be

harmful. The literature only mentions problems caused by excessively high blood calcium levels when values are between 150 and 200 ng/ml. 300 ng/ml and above is considered toxic (PMID:18689406).

Calculating the vitamin D dose for initial treatment: A single dose of 10,000 units is required to raise vitamin D levels by 1 ng/ml when body weight is 70 kg (154 lb). The dose is adjusted proportionately for other weights, because vitamin D is stored in all tissue, in fat, muscles and bones, as well as internal organs and body fluids. The greater the body mass, the more diluted the vitamin D consumed or formed through radiation, meaning its concentration in the blood is lower. The vitamin D dose must thus be increased accordingly. Practical clinical experience has confirmed this calculation method.

The upward deviation in vitamin D absorption and storage, which varies depending on the individual, is similarly kept within reasonable limits, so there is no risk of an overdose. The target value is reached with a fluctuation of ± 20 ng/ml.

Absorption can, however, be significantly, if not totally, blocked in patients with damaged intestinal mucosa. This results in an undersupply, and an alternative treatment may be necessary, e.g. through UVB radiation.

In some cases, patients may display poor vitamin D absorption without any visible signs or causes for this. It is thus an undersupply, rather than an overdose, which is a problem for some patients. This is why it is always advisable to conduct check-ups.

To dispel any fears about overdoses, we should remember that much higher doses were once commonplace in medicine: In the 1970s, every newborn was injected with 200,000 units (5 mg of Vigantol®) to prevent rickets. Infants were thus administered with up to 60,000 units per kilogram (meaning 25,000 per lbs) of body weight. In our initial vitamin D treatment, the one-off dose never exceeds 7,000 units per kilogram of body weight (meaning 3,000 per lbs), even in cases of extreme deficiency. That is just one eighth of the standard dose which was prescribed for infants in former times.

Calculating the vitamin D dose for ongoing treatment: The maintenance dose depends on the patient's body weight and on the target value. The monthly losses are between 10 and 30 percent. They may even be higher in smokers or people taking certain medications. The average loss is 20 percent.

Patients suffering from intestinal diseases and chronic diarrhea should undergo check-ups due to their impaired absorption, and their dose should be increased accordingly. In severe cases (e.g. Crohn's disease), vitamin D levels can be raised through injections or UVB radiation on the skin.

Based on these assumptions, a person with a normal weight of 70 kg (154 lb) needs 3,333 units a day (23,000 units a week) to achieve a vitamin D level of 50 ng/ml after an extended period of time.

For other body weights, the maintenance dose is adjusted proportionately using a correction factor. Double the weight thus requires double the dose, while half the weight requires half the dose. – The vitamin D content of food is negligible, and need not be taken into account when calculating the maintenance dose.

The vitamin D gained from sunbathing during the summer months increases vitamin D levels. It is safe to combine the maintenance treatment with sunbathing, because a target value of 50 ng/ml is around the lower limit of the optimum range, and vitamin D levels do not exceed 90 ng/ml even after extensive sun exposure. Critical values cannot be reached from the sun alone, even if vitamin D is already at an optimum level thanks to medication.

The maintenance treatment can, however, be temporarily paused if patients sunbathe intensively and generate a large amount of vitamin D.

Vitamin D dose for ongoing treatment of breastfeeding mothers: The study of Bruce Hollis has shown that breastfeeding mothers need at least 6,400 units a day in order to supply their infant with sufficient vitamin D. To be on the safe side, the infant can be given an additional 500 units orally per day. If the mother has a high body weight or is a smoker, a blood test can be performed to ensure the dose is increased if necessary, and the infant receives enough vitamin D.

For specialists: Individual calculation of parameters: The individual incremental factor can be calculated by retesting vitamin D levels after the one-off initial dose has been taken, and checking whether the target value has been reached. If there is a deviation from the calculated value, a correction factor must be calculated. This approach is particularly recommended for patients with intestinal disorders, who absorb less vitamin D. If the intestinal mucosa is found to be severely damaged, it may be necessary to chew the capsules, to take injections or UVB radiation.

The percentage absorption in the intestine improves with a low daily dose of less than 1,500 units. The incremental factor is higher in this case.

The loss rate is greater in smokers and persons who take certain medications (e.g. *carbamazepine* or *phenytoine*), as well as in breastfeeding mothers (increased loss through breast milk). The individual loss rate can also be calculated, which involves testing vitamin D levels one month after the initial treatment. Vitamin D supplements are then stopped for one to three months, before levels are checked again. A longer time frame reduces the effects of any errors when determining the loss rate. However, this method is only reliable during the winter months, when no vitamin D is gained through sunbathing. Consuming foods containing vitamin D does not usually skew results, unless the patient eats oily saltwater fish every day. To ensure the patient's vitamin D deficiency does not reoccur during this test, the initial value should be over 50 ng/ml.

Dosage limits for the vitamin D treatment

Nowadays high daily doses of 8,000 or 10,000 units are also being recommended. Whether or not this is a good idea depends on the individual case.

Body weight must be taken into account, and a distinction made between initial and ongoing treatment. If this is not done, vitamin D levels increase steadily. At a normal weight, an intake of 8,000 units a day, and a loss rate of 20 percent the level may exceed the recommended limit after one year.

Could it be that recommended doses are too high? Many studies did not take into account the participants' body weight. Therefore a person with a low weight will get a much higher vitamin D level. Today numerous participants are overweight. Vitamin D is thus spread over a greater body mass, and levels are lower than in thin people.

The high losses caused by smoking or taking certain medications may also skew test results. A high intake of vitamin D in such a person should not be transferred to a person without these factors.

Even with high daily doses, it takes well over a year to reach the equilibrium value, where supply and loss are balanced. Short-term studies conducted over a few weeks or months thus convey a false impression. People try to reach the target value in a short space of time through excessively high daily doses, without considering that this will push them over the target value in the long-term. A moderate overdose is not, however, dangerous, because the percentage vitamin D absorption is lower at high doses. To avoid misjudgments, a distinction must always be made between the one-off initial dose and the weekly maintenance dose.

During vitamin D treatment, laboratory tests should not be conducted straight after intake, as this will record high readings due to the rapid appearance of vitamin D in the blood. It is advisable to wait one to two months after the initial treatment, and three days after the weekly dose, to ensure blood levels match those in the cells (continue page 78).

On-off dose for initial treatment:

$$D_{IT} = (Vit.D_{TV} - Vit.D_C) \cdot CF_{BW} \cdot IF$$

Maintenance dose for ongoing treatment:

$$D_{OT} = Vit.D_{TV} \cdot LR \cdot CF_{BW} \cdot IF \qquad \textit{(per month)}$$

$$= (Vit.D_{TV} \cdot LR \cdot CF_{BW} \cdot IF) \cdot (7/30) \qquad \textit{(per week)}$$

$$= (Vit.D_{TV} \cdot LR \cdot CF_{BW} \cdot IF)/30 \qquad \textit{(per day)}$$

Legend:

D_{IT}	Dose for initial treatment [units]
D_{OT}	Dose for ongoing treatment [units]
$Vit.D_C$	Vitamin D level, current [ng/ml]
$Vit.D_{TV}$	Vitamin D level, target value [ng/ml]
IF	Incremental factor [10,000 units/(ng/ml)]
LR	Loss rate [0.2 = 20 percent per month]
CF_{BW}	Correction factor, body weight
$BW_{Pat.}$	Patient body weight [kg or lb]
BW_{Norm}	Normal body weight [70 kg or 154 lb]

$$CF_{BW} = \frac{BW_{Pat.}}{BW_{Norm}}$$

Formulae for calculating doses for the initial and ongoing treatment. The incremental factor and loss rate are average values, and vary in individual cases.

Short formula for initial treatment (capsules with 5,000 units): Number of capsules = Desired increase x body weight x 0.028
Example: 40 ng/ml x 100 kg x 0.028 = 112 capsules initially
Short formula for maintenance treatment (capsules per month): Number of capsules = Target value x body weight [kg] x 0.0056
Example: 50 ng/ml x 68 kg x 0.0056 = 19 capsules

Sample calculation 1

Patient body weight: 57 kg (126 lb)
Vitamin D level: 18 ng/ml
Vitamin D target value: 40 ng/ml

One-off dose for initial treatment:

$$= (40\text{-}18)\,\text{ng/ml}\ \frac{57\,\text{kg}}{70\,\text{kg}}\ \frac{10{,}000\,\text{units}}{1\,\text{ng/ml}}$$

= 180,000 units (first day 100,000 units and second day 80,000 units)

Maintenance dose for ongoing treatment:

$$= 40\,\text{ng/ml} \cdot 0{,}2 \cdot \frac{57\,\text{kg}}{70\,\text{kg}}\ \frac{10{,}000\,\text{units}}{1\,\text{ng/ml}}$$

= 65,000 units per month

Sample calculation 2

Patient body weight: 102 kg (225 lb)
Vitamin D level: 9 ng/ml
Vitamin D target value: 50 ng/ml

One-off dose for initial treatment:

$$= (50 - 9)\,\text{ng/ml}\ \frac{102\,\text{kg}}{70\,\text{kg}}\ \frac{10{,}000\,\text{units}}{1\,\text{ng/ml}}$$

= 600,000 units (100,000 units every six days)

Maintenance dose for ongoing treatment:

$$= 50\,\text{ng/ml} \cdot 0{,}2 \cdot \frac{102\,\text{kg}}{70\,\text{kg}}\ \frac{10{,}000\,\text{units}}{1\,\text{ng/ml}}$$

= 145,000 units per month

Sample calculations determining the dose of vitamin D for initial and ongoing treatment.

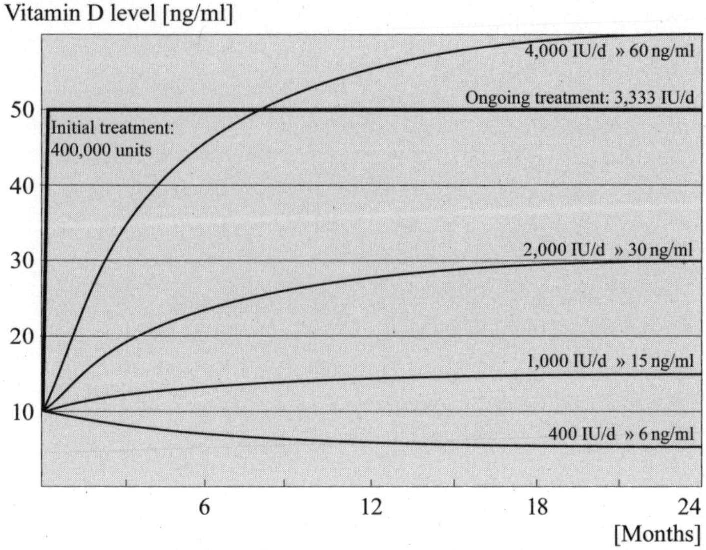

Vitamin D levels based on time, with varying vitamin D daily intake (parameter).

Assumptions: 1. Body weight: 70 kg (154 lb). – 2. Vitamin D level increased by 1 ng/ml with a one-off dose of 10,000 units. – 3. No vitamin D gained through UVB radiation on the skin. – 4. Vitamin D level drops by 20 percent a month. – 5. Initial value: 10 ng/ml. – 6. Target value: 50 ng/ml.

Calculation: The target value is reached within a few days of starting the initial treatment (one-off dose of 400,000 units), and is maintained with the ongoing treatment (3,333 units per day).

If a daily dose of 4,000 units is administered without performing the initial treatment, it will take four months until a level of 40 ng/ml is reached, and six months until 50 ng/ml is reached. The equilibrium value is 60 ng/ml. With a daily dose of 1,000 units, the equilibrium value is 15 ng/ml; so there is still a deficiency. With a daily dose of 400 units, the vitamin D level gradually drops to an equilibrium value of 6 ng/ml.

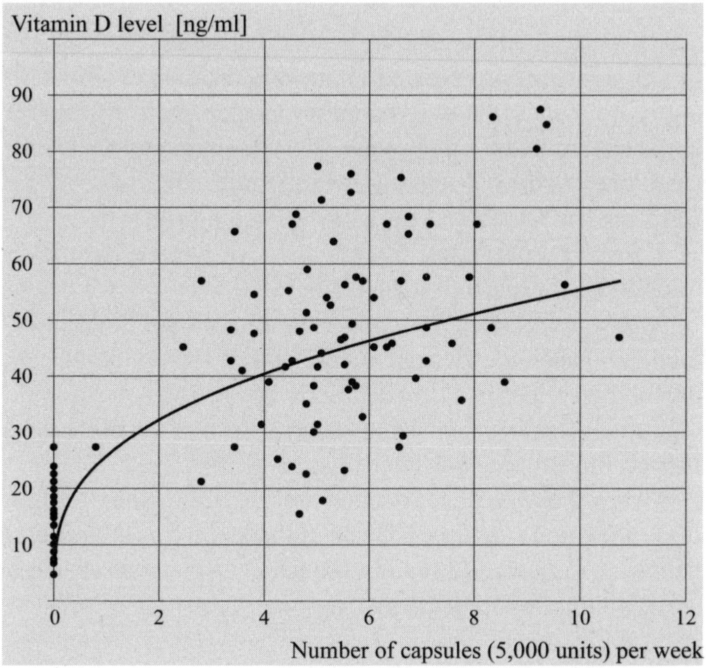

Vitamin D levels of various patients based on weekly maintenance dose, assuming a body weight of 70 kg (154 lb) (Institute Vitamindelta.de).

The graph shows the vast differences between patients even when the dose per kilogram of body weight remains the same. This high vertical deviation is due to the fact that absorption and loss rate vary in each individual.

There is no evidence that vitamin D levels are linearly dependent on the maintenance dose; the absorption rate drops significantly at higher doses. This effect means there is a reduced risk of overdosing.

On the far left are the data of those patients who did not receive any vitamin D medication over the winter.

Vitamin D medications

In Germany, all pre-formed vitamin D medications containing more than 1,000 units require a prescription. But this is a mistaken preventive measure. French pharmacies have for years been selling drinkable 200,000-unit ampoules on prescription for less than 2 Euros without any problems.

Capsules containing 50,000 units are freely available through mail ordering in the USA.

Many companies sell low-dose and liquid vitamin D medications on the German market under various names. As unpatented vitamin D medications are not very profitable, manufacturers have so far invested very little in marketing, though this attitude has been changing since 2011.

Given the high doses needed, tablet medications containing 1,000 units or less are not suitable for the vitamin D treatment, as it would require the patient to take an unnecessary amount of supplements.

Costs of vitamin D treatment

The initial treatment (e.g. 300,000 units in total) is not expensive and also the ongoing treatment is available at low cost. The treatment is thus not only effective and safe, but also extremely affordable.

Vitamin D levels only become critical when they exceed 150 ng/ml, because it is then that an unwanted calcium level can occur (hypercalcemia). In order to reach the critical threshold of 150 ng/ml, a patient weighing 70 kg (154 lb) would have to take a total of 1,500,000 units. As a precaution, the prescribed total dose should thus be less than this critical dose. This is still safe, even if the patient takes the whole content of the box.

The literature only mentions serious cases of poisoning for levels over 300 ng/ml. The safety margin between an optimum blood level and poisoning is thus greater than for most other medications.

Overdoses can only occur through miscalculation, or if the patient does not stick to the recommended doses. An older patient once particularly caught my attention when he asked for another prescription for his vitamin D medication just one month after starting the treatment. Upon questioning, I found out he had ignored the written instructions. After the initial treatment (300,000 units), he had taken another 700,000 units (20,000 a day). Despite this daily dose of 20,000 units, a check-up showed his vitamin D levels had only risen to 103 ng/ml. His calcium levels were normal, and he had no complaints. The ongoing treatment was suspended until his vitamin D levels dropped back to the target value, after which he resumed the maintenance dose.

In another case, having incorrectly taken 1,000,000 units over two weeks (80,000 units a day), a patient's vitamin D reached a level of 126 ng/ml. Her general condition and calcium levels were both normal.

The fear that vitamin D medications increase the risk of developing kidney stones has proven to be unfounded. The risk stated in former studies can be attributed on the additional use of calcium supplements. But with vitamin D no additional calcium is needed. Having issued thousands prescriptions myself, I personally have not found an elevated risk of kidney stones in patients taking vitamin D.

One thing is, however, worth explaining at this point. Calcium levels regularly rise to the upper normal range after the initial treatment. While many laboratories consider values over 2.60 mmol/l as abnormally high, international studies only classify readings of over 2.75 mmol/l as problematic "hypercalcemia" (abnormally high blood calcium levels). A group of researchers from Paris believes there is no risk if calcium levels remain below 3.00 mmol/l.

There are no sources describing risks for the 2.60 to 3.00 mmol/l range. The upper limit of 2.60 mmol/l merely reflects the consequences of the vitamin D deficiency. The fact that much of the world population is deficient means the dispersion range for vitamin D and calcium is lower. That is why it is necessary to normalize vitamin D levels without worrying about the "high" calcium levels, as long as these remain below 3.00 mmol/l. There is similarly no risk of the blood vessels "calcifying" as a result. It is rather the vitamin D deficiency which increases the risk of arteriosclerosis (literature references in the appendix).

If vitamin D levels are good, and diet is half-decent, calcium intake will be sufficient, so no medication is needed.

Flooding the body with calcium supplements can cause blood vessels to calcify, increasing the risk of heart attacks, strokes, and kidney damage. It is better to avoid calcium supplements, and to care for a nutrition which is rich in calcium and magnesium (especially vegetables) and to make sure that the vitamin D is at a good level.

Diet is important. Eating lots of highly acidic food (meat, cheese, curd, eggs, cereals) causes more calcium to be passed out in the sour urine. To prevent these losses, it is advisable to eat highly basic foods such as fruit, vegetables and potatoes. This is particularly crucial in old age, otherwise bone mass will degenerate to compensate for the increased calcium lost through the kidneys.

Salad and vegetables are also the foods with the highest calcium concentrations (the amount of calcium in relation to calories); even higher than milk. Fruit also has a relatively high content of calcium which is readily available to be resorbed. On the other hand, refined sugar, candy and flour products contain no or very little calcium, much like oils, fats and fatty foods. Wholegrain products also have a very low calcium concentration, and that little calcium is not readily available. Those wanting to improve their calcium intake and resorption thus simply need to eat more fruit and vegetables. At the same time their supply with other minerals, vitamins and antioxidants increases.

Nevertheless, a healthy diet and good vitamin D levels alone are not enough to prevent osteoporosis; the bones and muscles also need to be strengthened through regular training. Muscles and bones degenerate in equal measure if they are not used. Health-based strength training is the most effective way to build up muscle and bone. The elderly and even those needing care can gain muscle and bone mass by doing this. Strength training is the deciding factor.

Muscle training and vitamin D

Muscle training activates vitamin D, because calcium ions flow into the muscle cells to trigger a muscle contraction. This subtly reduces blood calcium levels, immediately prompting more stored vitamin D to be converted into its active form. More calcium is thus absorbed from the intestine, balancing out the calcium deficit in the blood.

After the muscle work, the active vitamin D then also performs its various genetic protective tasks in the cell and immune systems, which extend well beyond simply controlling the calcium metabolism. The active vitamin D has therefore been denoted as protectosterone (protecto meaning protection, and sterone meaning steroid hormone).

Muscle activity thus boosts the effectiveness of vitamin D by initially activating it, and the health-promoting effects of exercise and regular strength and endurance training are partly due to this.

Sufficient vitamin D levels are thus necessary to ensure optimum muscle and nerve function, which is why a deficiency leads to decreased muscle capacity, and an extreme deficiency can even cause muscle weakness and impaired co-ordination. Athletes in ancient times knew about this correlation instinctively, sunning themselves at every opportunity. This solar doping is safe, and results in many positive side effects.

All this shows how important it is to think holistically and incorporate all essential factors: sun, vitamin D levels, natural foods, sufficient exercise in everyday life, strength and endurance training, as well as good rest.

Treatment using UVB emitters

UVB radiation on the skin stimulates vitamin D formation. However, solarium lamps often only provide a small percentage of UVB, as they usually focus purely on achieving a quick tan through UVA radiation, reducing the amount of vitamin D produced. Penetrating deep into the skin, UVA radiation instead speeds up the skin ageing process, which is why frequent solarium visits should be enjoyed with caution. The glass in the tanning bed often filters out the desired UVB radiation, further decreasing the probability of generating vitamin D. Additionally, the longer the UV lamps are used, the weaker their UVB radiation becomes.

Special emitters have been developed to counteract these downsides. For example, the Osram Ultra Vitalux emitter contains a high percentage of UVB (about as much as that of a midday sun in the tropics). For seemingly liability-related reasons, however, these emitters are only sold by specialist retailers with the following warning: Not suitable for use on humans. So no one can officially recommend it for this purpose. The Ultra Vitalux emitter is therefore only used in equine solariums, and on iguanas, snakes and guinea pigs. People wishing to use these emitters need a heat-proof socket and mounting.

When UV radiation is performed at most solariums, neither the doctor nor the patient knows how much vitamin D is formed in each session. The UVB dose can differ greatly between the individual tanning beds. In unfavorable cases, a lot of radiation is performed and the patient looks nicely tanned, but vitamin D levels have barely increased, meaning deficiency cannot be rectified.

For this reason, patients should only visit certified solariums, where the equipment is guaranteed to provide an adequate amount of UVB.

The treatment using UVB emitters also takes a long time; several weeks even in the best case scenario, while medications can achieve optimum vitamin D levels within just a few days.

Before the skin is exposed to UV radiation, it is advisable to initially raise vitamin D levels through medication. This enables the skin to better tolerate the radiation.

Sunbathing

Sunbathing does a lot more than just stimulate vitamin D production. You only have to think about the beneficial heat emitted and the bright daylight, which promotes wellbeing. That's why every sunny day should be taken advantage of to soak up a hefty dose of sun, without stressing the skin by overdosing on UV radiation.

Unfortunately, in the northern countries (above 40 degrees latitude) sunbathing only provides vitamin D during the summer months. No UVB radiation reaches the earth's surface between October and March, because the rays from the low-sitting sun have to cover a long distance through the atmosphere, and are filtered out. Only when the sun is at least 45 degrees above the horizon, i.e. when an object is larger than its shadow, is UVB radiation intense enough to effectively stimulate vitamin D production.

When the sky is gloriously blue (clear air and therefore intense UVB radiation), even the lowly positioned sun is, however, enough to warrant sunbathing to generate some vitamin D. These days should be taken advantage of.

For example in Germany, radiation is better in the southern than in the northern part. Intensity is at its peak in the high altitudes of the Alps in the south. The same difference exists in other countries with a large north-south extension, like France or the UK, and especially in large countries like the USA, Australia or Russia.

On the other hand, haze and polluted air, particularly in big cities, reduce UVB radiation, thereby prolonging the winter period in which no vitamin D can be produced.

UVB radiation is also weather-dependent. If it is cloudy, vitamin D cannot be produced, even in summer.

As UVB radiation reaches its daily peak when the sun is at its highest position, the time around noon should be used for sunbathing. The solar noon depends on location; one hour is added due to daylight saving. Even in the middle of summer, hardly any vitamin D can be produced before 9am and after 4pm.

But the best sunny conditions are pointless if you cannot go outside and sunbathe at noon due to work, school or household duties. Office workers in tropical countries still have vitamin D deficiency because they have to spend their entire working day in closed rooms.

There is similarly no point in only exposing your face, hands and forearms to the midday sun, while the rest of the body is covered up. In this case, the amount of skin exposed to the radiation is often too little to raise vitamin D levels. Only by sunning the entire body can 10,000 to 20,000 units of vitamin D be absorbed per day.

All sunscreens seek to block UVB radiation and thus prevent vitamin D from forming. They should only be used if the skin cannot be protected from excessive UV radiation by staying in the shade or covering up.

Another problem lies in the fact that many people can no longer tolerate the intense UV radiation, and thus avoid the midday sun. This is usually due to the skin not having had the chance to adjust to the sun. Pigmentation and skin hardening (light-induced callosity) take time. When a vitamin D deficiency is present, the skin is more sensitive to UV rays, making sun-based treatment more difficult, and meaning longer acclimatization periods are required.

An incorrect diet makes the skin susceptible to sunburn, particularly if it lacks antioxidants, such as vitamin C, carotene and carotenoids, which are found in fruit and vegetables. This also impedes sun therapy, especially for patients with severe vitamin D deficiency, even though they so desperately need sun.

Unfortunately, this sort of treatment additionally only works in fine weather, and even then it is long drawn-out. With intensive UVB radiation and full body exposure to the sun, up to 20,000 units of vitamin D can be produced every day. Twenty of such sunny days would be needed, i.e. three weeks of perfect sunshine and summer weather, to rectify a typical deficiency with 400,000 units.

With changeable weather, haze and family commitments, most people would need two whole months of summer to achieve this. And this does not include the time required for the skin to grow accustomed to the sun. In some cases, the summer is already over before good vitamin D levels can even be reached, and then they drop back straight away.

Those lucky enough to spend ten summer days under a glorious blue sky (high UVB intensity) and sun their entire body while on vacation will achieve around 200,000 units of vitamin D. If, upon returning from vacation, they are back in the office or factory from 8am to 4pm without stocking up on vitamin D, this considerable gain will be lost after just two months. Occasional weekend sunbathing does not help much. This shows how hard it is to maintain good vitamin D levels purely through sunbathing when working a regular eight-hour day.

Sun therapy was previously practiced predominantly in the Alps, whose high altitude, clear air and southerly location provided more intense UVB radiation compared to the lowlands. But even there, patients were limited to the months between February and October, and were dependent on fine weather. Altitude treatment at that time took at least two to three months.

Those wanting to undergo sun therapy in winter nowadays have to travel to the far South. At the time of the winter solstice four weeks are needed. A short break only results in a slight increase in vitamin D levels.

Sun therapy is thus a long drawn-out affair. If optimum vitamin D levels cannot be reached through sunbathing alone, they should be raised through medication. The ideal scenario would be to ensure a basic intake through medication, plus use every opportunity to soak up some well-dosed sun.

The advantages of treating vitamin D deficiency with medication

Vitamin D deficiency can be rectified quickly and effectively with medication, regardless of location, weather or season. Even patients who are not physically or mentally able to gain vitamin D through sunbathing, e.g. the ill, the disabled, and those requiring care, can be treated. All those whose professional, school and domestic commitments prevent them from finding time to sunbathe at noon can be helped. Those who do not have the time or money to travel to the sunny South in winter can rectify their vitamin D deficiency with medication.

The fastest, most effective way to treat illnesses caused by vitamin D deficiency is to take vitamin D supplements.

Vitamin D is also essential for preventing acute and chronic diseases, particularly in winter.

Vitamin D content in food

Most foods contain no, or only traces of, vitamin D. Even saltwater fish does little to boost vitamin D levels, which is why hardly any vitamin D is absorbed through food.

Very few types of fish are high in vitamin D. These are herring, salmon and eel (see table). But this is only the case for wild fish. Contrary to a mistaken belief, fish cannot produce vitamin D themselves. The vitamin D found in fish comes from certain specialized species of tropical plankton, which use vitamin D to protect their genes from the intense UV rays of the tropical sun. That is, because the nucleic acids and vitamin D have the same molecular resonance frequency.

Vitamin D reaches the europaen shores in the the form of plankton – through sea currents (gulf stream) and fish migration. The vitamin D content in saltwater fish is thus also dependent on the place it is caught. Most freshwater fish contain no vitamin D, and the vitamin D content in fish from aquafarms is similarly overestimated, as they often receive little vitamin D from their food.

Grilling and frying destroys half the vitamin D, in some cases up to 95 percent. Fried fish therefore cannot meet the body's vitamin D requirements, even if kilos of it are eaten. Consuming raw fish, on the other hand, involves the risk of infection through nematodes and other parasites.

Fish are often charged with environmental pollutants, which is why it is not advisable to eat large quantities regularly. The same is true for cod liver oil, which comes from the liver of the cod and haddock.

Vitamin D	Content Units / 100 g	Vitamin D	Content Units / 100 g
Breast milk	0,5–5	Herring	1080
Milk (3.5 % fat)	2–5	Salmon	640–880
Yoghurt (3.5 % fat)	2–3	Eel	840
Curd (40 % fat)	8	Sardines	400
Butter	10–50	Trout	280
Cream	45	Tuna	240
Edam Cheese	12	Cod	40
Emmental Cheese	45	Mackerel	40
Gorgonzola	40	Cod liver oil	12000
Avocado	140–200	Beef liver	68
Mushroom	80	Pork liver	40
Hen's egg	50–120	Margarine	10–40

Vitamin D content of certain foods.

The vitamin D content of milk, eggs and meat depends on how much vitamin D the animals have been able to produce in the sun and absorb through food. Vitamin D synthesis is not possible in animals kept in barns. Between 50 and 100 units of vitamin D per 100 grams are usually added to the feed.

Since 50 to 95 percent of vitamin D is destroyed through frying, the stated values must be reduced accordingly in cases of fried food.

The low vitamin D content in human breast milk is due to the fact that most breastfeeding mothers suffer from severe vitamin D deficiency without even realizing it. A mother needs around 6,400 units a day to provide her infant with sufficient vitamin D.

Avocado is a useful source of vitamin D, though it can still only cover a small part of the body's overall requirement.

Cod liver oil is high in vitamin D, but unfortunately also very high in vitamin A. Reaching and maintaining optimum levels of vitamin D would require eating vast quantities, which would soon result in vitamin A poisoning. Cod liver oil is thus not suitable as a vitamin D supplement. In earlier times, when no medication was available, it was considered an acceptable way of preventing and treating rickets.

Cod liver oil also tastes foul, originating from the rancid fats caused by the oxidation of highly unsaturated fatty acids during straining and storage. This means that an oil of bad taste is not only inedible, but also toxic – another reason to substitute it with vitamin D medication.

The vitamin D content of milk, cheese and butter is low, and depends on whether or not the dairy cow lives on grazing land and produces vitamin D in the sun. Winter, when vitamin D requirements are at their highest, is precisely when milk and dairy products contain only traces of vitamin D, doing nearly nothing to boost levels.

Margarine contains minimal vitamin D, meaning that even excessive consumption fails to meet the body's requirements. Food advertising for 100 units of vitamin D is equally misleading, since all varieties contain negligible amounts.

Correct sunbathing with high gain of vitamin D

In order to achieve a high vitamin D synthesis when sunbathing, and not damage your skin by overdosing on UV radiation, the following principles must be followed:

- Expose a large area of skin to the sun, ideally the entire body on both sides.
- The sun's rays should hit the skin at a vertical angle wherever possible, maximizing the vitamin D synthesized.
- The ideal time is noon, when the sun is at its highest (specifically solar noon, which depends on location; the one-hour difference during summer must be taken into account). The higher the sun, the more intense the UVB radiation, and the more UVB is absorbed. Large quantities of vitamin D are produced when the sun is at a high position over 45°.
- Sunbathe at noon on every sunny day, even if it's only for a few minutes.
- Sunny days with a gloriously blue sky are perfect, because UVB radiation is most intense when air is clear.
- The only way to sun yourself when inside is through an open window. Window glass blocks UVB radiation, though you can still get sunburnt from UVA radiation.
- Avoid excess. The first few minutes of sunbathing are the most valuable. Vitamin D production decreases with every minute, because the UV radiation consumes the precursors of vitamin D. After a while, an equilibrium

value is reached, and no more vitamin D can be produced. Spending a long time sunbathing is pointless and will only damage the skin. Even with tanned skin, a large amount of vitamin D can be produced in just half an hour (15 minutes lying on stomach, and 15 minutes lying on back) if radiation conditions are good.
It is advisable to follow my „clock-face rule“ when UV radiation is intense (noon at the beach in the Mediterranean, with clear blue skies), especially if skin has not yet adapted to the sun's rays:
Skin type 1: 5 minutes each lying on back and stomach.
Skin type 2: 10 minutes each (clock-face 2).
Skin type 3: 15 minutes each (clock-face 3).
Skin type 4: 20 minutes each etc. (clock-face 4 etc.).
The ideal duration for sunbathing in peak summer can be extended by 5 minutes; the times must be doubled (but no more than tripled) when sunbathing in the morning or afternoon, or in spring or late summer.

- Allow the skin to gradually adapt to the sun. It should be exposed to no more than half the sunburn time (M. Holick's rule), which is the time frame after which the skin starts to redden. The skin's own light protection factor can be increased to 40 (for skin types 3 and 4) through pigmentation and hardening.
- Eating lots of fruit and vegetables allows the skin to better tolerate UV rays (particularly through carotene, carotenoids, vitamin C and E, as well as other antioxidants).
- The skin can create its own suitable light protection through a healthy diet and adaptation to the sun, meaning no sunscreens are required for everyday activities or intense sunbathing.

- The skin must have a sufficiently high concentration of vitamin D, boosted by medication if necessary. This cures many sun allergies.
- Do not put any sunscreen when you start the radiation. This blocks UVB rays and almost totally prevents vitamin D production.
- If you are extensively exposed to the sun, the skin must be covered up under clothing. Any necessary cream should only be put on the exposed areas, such as face and hands. Preference should be given to creams containing mineral UV protection.

Depending on lifetime exposure, sun damage is primarily caused by UVA radiation, which penetrates deep into the skin. Optimum radiation thus means evenly exposing the entire body's skin to the necessary amount of UVB radiation, thereby also keeping UVA radiation within acceptable limits. Sunbathing sessions should therefore be spread over as many days as possible, and take place in the noon sun.

A high UVB-UVA ratio is achieved by:

- The sun being in a high position (over 45°).
- Clear air (bright blue sky) – no clouds, haze, dust or air pollutants.
- Refraining from using sunscreens (reduces UVB radiation to just a few percent, depending on light protection factor, quantity used, and re-applications).
- Not sunbathing behind window glass. Glass completely filters out UVB radiation.
- Ideally lying down when sunbathing. When standing up, you are exposed to greater UVA radiation through reflection. The UVB rays are hardly reflected, but instead largely absorbed. Radiation levels in snowy and icy

conditions in high-altitude mountains (at glaciers and ski slopes), on the water (when sailing and canoeing), on white sand, and on concrete are critical, which is why sunbathing at the beach, on the balcony, or on the terrace is less recommended. The reflected UVA radiation is minimized at the beach by lying flat on the sand. A much better option would be to sunbathe amongst green nature, because the chlorophyll in the leaves absorbs the UVA rays (only the green, visible light is reflected). When sunbathing in the garden, you are thus only exposed to the direct rays containing a high amount of UVB, which is ideal for skin.

- Tanning beds with intense UVA radiation and low UVB radiation should be avoided. Only certified equipment providing an improved percentage of UVB radiation, equivalent to that of a high midday sun or tropical sun, is acceptable.

Those who follow these principles will gain lots of vitamin D through UVB radiation and minimize the stress on their skin caused by UVA radiation, thereby keeping UV-based skin ageing within reasonable limits.

The face should be spared when sunbathing, particularly as it is already exposed to the most UV. Prematurely aged facial skin resulting from excessive UVA radiation cannot be concealed. That's why it is advisable to sun the back more and keep the face out of the sun, or protect it from excessive radiation using a hat.

If this method is applied, and every sunny day is used for midday sunbathing, optimum vitamin D levels can even be achieved in northern countries like Canada, Ireland, Great Britain, the Netherlands, Germany and Denmark, from spring through to fall. And when the wintertime comes, vitamin D medications can help people benefit from their protective effects all year round.

Concerns over vitamin D

Concerns over treating a vitamin D deficiency often arise if a patient is already chronically ill and anxiously reads the package insert. Older package inserts in particular are more about protecting the manufacturer from possible claims rather than providing a statistical description of the actual risks.

Recurring questions from everyday practice are only answered briefly here, as a full scientific discussion would go beyond the scope of this book. By visiting the freely accessible website www.pubmed.gov, you can use the keywords mentioned here to access the latest scientific discussions.

Intolerance reactions are rare, and are most likely due to one of the carrier substances in some vitamin D medications. In this case, a different supplement should be taken.

Vitamin D taken orally is better than injections

Taking a one-off dose of 100,000 units causes vitamin D levels to peak around five days later (PMID: 18326608), while a higher dose involves a later peak. No check-ups should thus be performed for at least a week; and for higher doses at least a month.

If injected into the muscles, vitamin D takes weeks or months to be released and spread around the body (PMID 18492750). If the effective level needs to be checked, this should only be done after a month in order to avoid misinterpretations.

Calcium medication

Is it necessary to take additional calcium supplements? Although a high-dose calcium intake had shown beneficial effects in a population with vitamin D defiency, it should be left to the body's own regulatory system once vitamin D levels have been normalized. Taking calcium consistently over the long term poses several health risks, and suppresses vitamin D activation.

Pubmed.gov: vitamin d calcium adverse

Embryonic phase

Can a woman take vitamin D when pregnant? Tests on hens have shown that a lack of vitamin D in food results in serious deformities and the death of embryos. On the other hand, these problems disappear when vitamin D is administered (PMID: 5401066). Vitamin D is thus considered a protective factor for embryos.

Pubmed.gov: vitamin d teratogenicity

Pregnancy

Can taking vitamin D affect a pregnancy? The study conducted by Bruce Hollis showed that a daily dose of vitamin D during pregnancy reduces all typical risks. There are fewer Cesareans and fewer complications when women take 6,400 units a day.

Pubmed.gov: vitamin d pregnancy Hollis B

Breastfeeding

How does vitamin D intake impact on a breastfed infant? Bruce Hollis showed that breast milk only contained enough vitamin D for the infant when a dose of at least 6,400 units was administered. This provides additional protection for the child's development.

Pubmed.gov: vitamin d lactation

Childhood

What do we need to remember when it comes to children? Children have thinner skin and can thus produce vitamin D very quickly between April and September. If no optimum vitamin D level can be reached from the sun, medications should be taken. Capsules, however, are not a good idea, because they can get into the airways, particularly in smaller children. Oily vitamin D supplements with direct oral application should be prefered. It would be a mistake to add drops of this oily medication to a glass of water, because the oil will stick to the side of the glass.

In former times 200,000 units used to be the standard prophylaxis to prevent rickets in newborn babies.

Pubmed.gov: vitamin d children supplementation

The elderly

What do we need to remember when over 60? A dose of 100,000 units administered every four months reduces the bone breakages. Within a three-year period, only 6 instead of 8 per cent of patients will suffer from fractures (PMID: 12609940).

However, it is not a good idea to take a high vitamin D dose as a one off and then nothing at all, because vitamin D levels will end up dropping again. Low levels presumably prevent motor nerve cells from functioning properly (W. STUMPF), which has a negative impact on the muscles' coordination capacity. The fracture rate thus increases when a single dose of 300,000 units is taken only every four months. The rise and fall of the vitamin D level is even more pronounced if a dose of 500,000 units is taken once a year (PMID: 17998225 and 20460620). To avoid this, it is not only necessary to reach an optimum vitamin D level (initial treatment), but also maintain this with constant intake (maintenance treatment). Mini doses are just as useless as mega doses taken every few months or once a year.

Diabetes

What can diabetics expect? Vitamin D improves the glucose regulation. During pregnancy, vitamin D reduces the risk of diabetes, while in children, it drastically reduces the risk of developing type I diabetes. In some cases, incipient type I diabetes was found to go into remission.

Pubmed.gov: vitamin d diabetes mellitus

Lung diseases

Should people with poor lung function be treated with vitamin D? There is significant evidence of vitamin D's special protective function when it comes to lung disease and COPD (*Chronic Obstructive Pulmonary Disease* – reduced lung function; PMID: 21419281). Vitamin D can thus certainly be recommended in such cases.

Pubmed.gov: Vitamin D COPD

Calcified blood vessels

Are there risks associated with taking vitamin D medication if blood vessel calcification is present? Arteriosclerotic processes may be inhibited.

Pubmed.gov: vitamin d arteriosclerosis

Hypercalcemia

What should you do if high blood calcium levels of over 2.60 mmol/l are recorded before or during treatment?

Due to the worldwide undersupply of vitamin D, the distribution curve for blood calcium levels has dropped to a lower level. It is a different story in sunnier countries, where 2.75 to 3.00 mmol/l are classified as the upper limits (PMID: 20398761).

True hypercalcemia, with values of over 3.00 mmol/l, does not even occur when vitamin D treatment is administered over the long-term. Values below this level are considered to be harmless.

Pubmed.gov: vitamin d hypercalcaemia mmol/l

Thrombosis risk

Does the risk of thrombosis increase when you take vitamin D medication? No, the risks of thrombosis will most likely drop when vitamin D reaches an optimum level (PMID: 20886515).

Heart diseases

Should people with poor cardiac muscle function be treated? There is significant evidence of vitamin D's ability to protect people with heart disease. It must be recommended, as it reduces mortality (PMID: 18635847).

Pubmed.gov: vitamin d heart failure

Dementia

What happens with dementia patients? It has a positive effect.

Pubmed.gov: vitamin d dementia

Kidney stones

Does vitamin D medication increase the risk of kidney stones? No, studies of over 100,000 participants have shown it to be safe (PMID: 20486209).

Renal insufficiency

Should people with poor kidney function be treated? There is a lot of evidence to show that vitamin D provides particular protection for people with kidney disease. It should thus be recommended.

Pubmed.gov: vitamin d chronic kidney disease

Abnormal release of parathormone

Is it possible to have an abnormal increase in blood calcium levels? The study conducted by J R Tucci showed that, despite excessive parathormone activity, the feared hypercalcemia did not occur after a high dose of vitamin D. In contrast, primary and secondary hyperparathyroidism always normalized when vitamin D was taken (PMID: 19383807 and 2152424).

Sarcoidosis

What happens if someone with undetected sarcoidosis takes vitamin D? When taking vitamin D, it is possible for hypercalcemia to occur if there is active sarcoidosis, which is a very rare condition, indicated by an elevated ACE serum level. If, however, slowly increasing doses of vitamin D are applied, it can unexpectedly cure long-time sarcoidosis. The body presumably needs vitamin D to control defective cells. (RAIMUND VON HELDEN: *Anticancer Research, Vitamin D Symposium*. May 2011, conference in Bad Homburg.)

Daytime vitamin D activation cycle

The conversion of stored vitamin D into its active form increases in the morning based on physical activity, reaching its daily maximum at midday, dropping slightly during early afternoon siestas, increasing again later in the afternoon, declining somewhat in the evening, and dropping sharply later at night. The concentration of active vitamin D reaches its lowest point between midnight and getting up the next morning (PMID: 11980618). All in all the rise and fall of the active form of vitamin D reflects the muscular activity.

Appendix: GP observations
Dr. Raimund von Helden's Praxis

Rapid improvement in dysautonomia through vitamin D

Background: Many everyday symptoms, such as adynamia, listlessness, chronic fatigue, rapid exhaustion, circulatory complaints, sleeping disorders, leg pain, calf cramps, muscle twitches, eyelid twitches, headaches, foot pain and back pain, often cannot be explained, despite extensive examinations. If no organic causes can be found, the most common diagnosis is "dysautonomia/autonomic dysfunction", or nervous system dysfunction. The term autonomic means that this part of the nervous system works involuntarily. We are familiar with this from things such as blood pressure, heartbeat and breathing rate. It is believed that a dysfunctional nervous system may be due to a calcium deficiency, which is in turn caused by a vitamin D deficiency.

This gave rise to the idea to check the extent to which patients with a serious vitamin D deficiency and dysautonomia noticed an improvement when vitamin D levels were increased.

Patients: 228 patients aged between 13 and 87 had a vitamin D deficiency. They were given an initial dose to raise their levels to between 40 and 60 ng/ml, and then received a maintenance dose.

Method: The vitamin D dose for the initial and maintenance treatment was calculated based on the rules described in this book.

The dose for the initial treatment was split into several daily doses of 100,000 units. A maintenance dose of a minimum 20,000 units per week was then prescribed. The patients were asked to complete a questionnaire, giving their personal rating of the treatment's benefits, from „zero stars" (no improvement) to „five stars" (fully cured):

Results: 78 percent of the ratings submitted within the first seven days showed positive results; 45 percent of the patients rated the vitamin D treatment with four or five stars (see overview on the next page).

Conclusion: The observations made during this study confirmed the hypothesis that a vitamin D deficiency is a common and significant cause of dysautonomia. Around four fifths of the patients benefited from having their vitamin D levels raised. The positive results are usually achieved very quickly. No seriously adverse effects were recorded.

Given that vitamin D deficiency is so common in the northern countries, and chronic autonomic symptoms are so widespread, correct vitamin D treatment provides great benefits at low cost, with no risks, and the bonus of having a preventive capacity. Vitamin D treatment should thus always be considered for dysautonomia patients.

Ratings by 228 patients after an average of 17 days

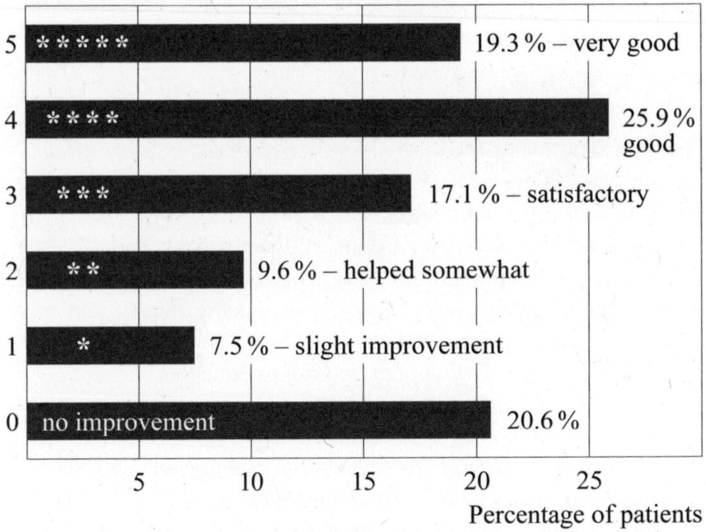

Ratings by 228 dysautonomia patients regarding the benefits of vitamin D treatment (for more information, www.vitamin-Delta.de/studie.html).

Just under half the patients (45 percent) rated the treatment as “good” or “very good”. Almost two thirds (62 percent) deemed it “satisfactory” to “very good”. These improvements turned out to be permanent.

Only 20 percent of patients found there to be no improvement. No one complained that their condition had worsened, and that is no surprise, since vitamin D is non-toxic and essential to life.

Literature

HELDEN, RAIMUND VON: *Vitamin-D-Lehrgang*. pdf-file. www.VitaminDelta.de (2011).

HOLICK, MICHAEL; JENKINS, MARK: *Schützendes Sonnenlicht*. Stuttgart 2005.

HOLICK, MICHAEL: *The Vitamin D Solution: A 3-Step Strategy to Cure Our Most Common Health Problems*. New York 2010.

KLEIN, THOMAS: *Sonnenlicht, das größte Gesundheitsgeheimnis. Sonnenmangel und seine schwerwiegenden Folgen.* 2nd edition Dresden 2010.

SORENSON, MARC: *Vitamin D3 and Solar Power for optimal Health*. 2nd edition Saint George 2008.

SPITZ, JÖRG: *Vitamin D. Das Sonnenhormon für unsere Gesundheit und der Schlüssel zur Prävention.* Schlangenbad 2008.

SPITZ, JÖRG; GRANT, WILLIAM: *Krebszellen mögen keine Sonne.* Lünen 2009.

WORM, NICOLAI: *Heilkraft D.* Lünen 2009.

ZITTERMANN, ARMIN: *Vitamin D in der Präventivmedizin.* Bremen 2010.

Index